Apple Cider Vinegar
HANDBOOK

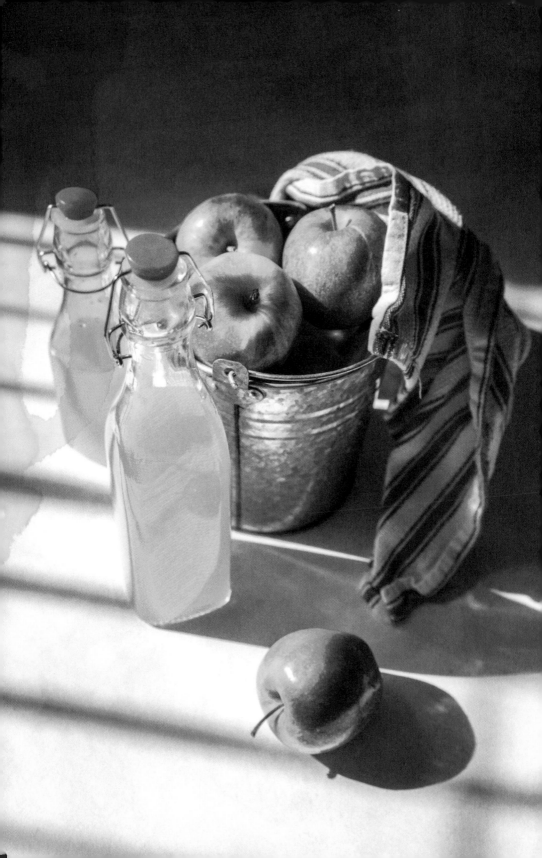

Recipes for **Natural Living**

Apple Cider Vinegar
HANDBOOK

AMY LEIGH MERCREE

Foreword by Kac Young, PhD

STERLING
New York

STERLING

New York

An Imprint of Sterling Publishing Co., Inc.
1166 Avenue of the Americas
New York, NY 10036

ISBN 978-1-4549-2897-3

Library of Congress Cataloging-in-Publication Data
Names: Mercree, Amy Leigh, author.
Title: Apple cider vinegar handbook : recipes for natural living / Amy
   Leigh Mercree.
Description: New York, NY : Sterling Publishing Co., Inc., [2018] | Includes
   bibliographical references.
Identifiers: LCCN 2018000116 (print) | LCCN 2018002289 (ebook) | ISBN
   9781454929116 (e-book) | ISBN 9781454928973 (paperback)
Subjects: LCSH: Cider vinegar--Therapeutic use--Popular works. | Cider
   vinegar--Health aspects--Popular works. | BISAC: HEALTH & FITNESS /
   Healthy Living.
Classification: LCC RM666.V55 (ebook) | LCC RM666.V55 M47 2018 (print) |
DDC
   615.3/23642--dc23
LC record available at
https://lccn.loc.gov/2018000116

Distributed in Canada by Sterling Publishing Co., Inc.
c/o Canadian Manda Group, 664 Annette Street
Toronto, Ontario M6S 2C8, Canada
Distributed in the United Kingdom by GMC Distribution Services
Castle Place, 166 High Street, Lewes, East Sussex BN7 1XU, England
Distributed in Australia by NewSouth Books
45 Beach Street, Coogee, NSW 2034, Australia

For information about custom editions, special sales, and premium and corporate purchases,
please contact Sterling Special Sales at 800-805-5489 or specialsales@sterlingpublishing.com.

Manufactured in the United States of America

2 4 6 8 10 9 7 5 3 1

sterlingpublishing.com

Cover design by Elizabeth Mihaltse Lindy
Interior design by Christine Heun
For picture credits see page 218

CONTENTS

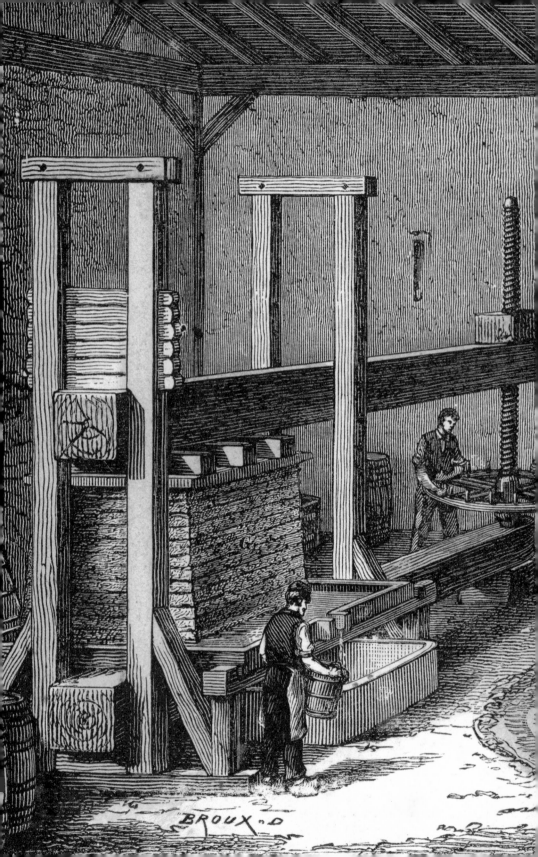

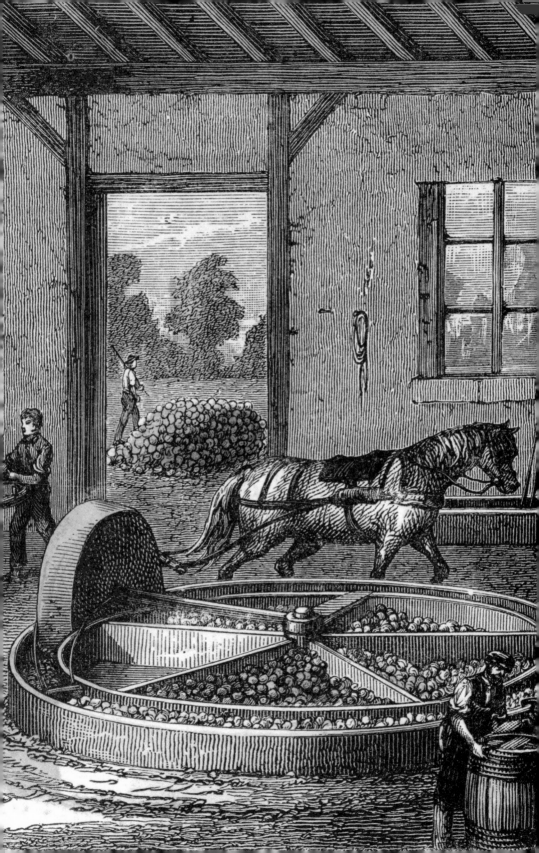

FOREWORD

Apple Cider Vinegar Handbook is an information-packed resource by Amy Leigh Mercree featuring the multiple health benefits of apple cider vinegar (ACV). Ms. Mercree leads us on a captivating journey, showing us how to enhance our natural bodily systems, resulting in a healthier physique, by incorporating ACV as a regular part of our food intake.

As I write this, I am sipping on Ms. Mercree's wonderful recipe for Roman *posca* (chapter 1), which may be one of the most interesting and delicious drinks I have ever imbibed. I was not unfamiliar with the use of ACV, but Ms. Mercree has expanded and extended those uses into a resourceful book that is as easily digested as ACV.

ACV may be one of the best hidden treasures of the world, and Ms. Mercree, with her background in healing and counseling, might just be another.

In *Apple Cider Vinegar Handbook*, Ms. Mercree educates us with her lavish knowledge of ACV, treats us to a fascinating history of it, the various methods used in fermentation, and why a particular method enhances ACV's health benefits.

The common complaints I hear regularly in my naturopathic and hypnotherapy practice are overall health concerns: loss of energy, the need for weight reduction or smoking cessation, the desire for longevity, recurring conditions, and chronic pain. I have been a longtime advocate that food either heals us or hurts us; every bite we take either fights disease or feeds it.

These familiar grievances are conditions caused, or exacerbated by, inflammation (heart disease, arthritis, diabetes, obesity), weight management (diet, exercise, anorexia), and gut health and digestion (acidity, heartburn, indigestion, frequent colds, IBS, stomach upset, immune disorders). Ms. Mercree's book discusses many of these root causes and suggests cures for them through the use of ACV.

In my practice, I find that a majority of my clients come to me because they are constantly plagued by weight challenges. Some can't seem to keep the weight off; others don't want to eat at all and are dangerously underweight. Weight control is a source of deep emotional stress for them as well as being the main culprit in many of their related health concerns. I believe Ms. Mercree's easy-to-read book will improve my clients' understanding of the chemistry of their bodies and how they can use ACV to help regulate key physical processes.

According to Ms. Mercree, ACV taken regularly can affect metabolism and stimulate gastric acids to assist the body in digesting food and eliminating waste. She even suggests that ACV can help cure the ordinary cold, or at the very least, reduce its symptoms and shorten the life of the bacteria or virus causing the discomfort.

Ms. Mercree skillfully walks us through a myriad of common complaints throughout her well-organized chapters and explains how ACV can aid in alleviating many common ills. Her description of the acid-alkaline balance is clear and right on the mark. In my practice I emphasize that the key to proper digestion is the intricate balance of alkaline and acid foods in the system. Too much of one or the other hampers effective digestion and the subsequent absorption of minerals and vitamins into the bloodstream from the foods we eat and drink.

If we keep our body at an even pH (power of hydrogen) balance, many of our complaints naturally disappear. Our ideal pH is slightly alkaline: 7.30 to 7.45. When we regulate our body's balance, we allow it to function at a higher level, since it is not required to waste vital energy removing acids and toxins in a frantic attempt to rebalance a pH that is off-kilter. Ms. Mercree stresses that AVC helps the body to stay in acidic-alkaline balance, thereby improving our health and energy. The chart she provides in chapter 3 thoroughly explains what a body should be consuming for optimal pH balance. That chart alone is worth the price of the book.

In her book, Ms. Mercree clearly explains that vinegar is, at its core, acetic acid. This beneficial acid is composed of necessary proteins, enzymes, probiotics, phosphorous, magnesium, potassium, and calcium. It is not like any other vinegar since it comes from the fermented juice of an apple and, similar to kombucha, forms a SCOBY layer (that is, a symbiotic culture of bacteria and yeast), which holds the nutrients and minerals that assist the body in multiple functions.

ACV also helps regulate blood sugar. In a study from Arizona State University, subjects took a drink of 20 grams of apple cider vinegar, 40 grams of water, and 1 teaspoon of artificial sweetener with each meal. Those with insulin resistance who drank the vinegar had 34 percent lower postprandial (after-meal) glucose compared to controls.

A key factor in overall physical health is the amount of toxins and free radicals the body is required to process and flush. Extra stress on the kidneys and liver can result in several life-threatening hazards from renal failure to dialysis, heart disease, and lupus. Chapter 4 details the process of detox and how that alone can readily assist a person with weight loss. Ms. Mercree writes, "Effective detoxification can kick this process into high gear. Along with whole, unprocessed foods, one of the simplest items in your weight management/detox arsenal is ACV."

She describes the need for detoxification to rid the body of dangerous toxins, which are stored in fat deposits, the liver, the lymph nodes, the lungs, the skin, and other organs, thus freeing these organs from the burden of processing ingested toxins and free radicals we put into the body from food, chemical, smog, and environmental contaminants.

My work with essential oils makes inclusion of ACV a comfortable addition to my recommendations for clients to improve their health and well-being. Ms. Mercree highlights the need for proper dilution and the correct doses and handling of ACV. The same is true for essential oils, and I admire her repetition of the cautions to avoid using ACV internally full strength. Dilution stands to reason because, used full strength, ACV is also an effective rust preventive, counter cleaner, wart antidote, natural food preservative, and fungus inhibitor.

In my work, I judge things by my personal scale of SARO: Is it sensible, achievable, and result-oriented? If it is, then I adopt it. Ms. Mercree's book is certainly that and more. She has included dozens of original recipes to help get readers started on integrating ACV into their wellness plan. I will be enjoying her hummus and guacamole recipes this very weekend with my family.

By following Amy Mercree's well-researched engaging style, and knowledgeable suggestions, I truly believe we could improve our inner and outer health and improve our physical image simultaneously. I have already begun to think of new ways to incorporate ACV in my recommendations for clients, and most certainly I will encourage them to make use of this fine presentation and well-written book.

—KAC YOUNG, PhD, ND, DCH

Ventura, California

INTRODUCTION

My earliest memory of vinegar is from early childhood. My yiayia, Dora, always made oil and vinegar salad dressing, and she went heavy on the vinegar. Its tart flavor would fill your senses. Its smell and taste were distinct and still remind me of our Greek Easter and New Year's Day celebrations.

Several times a year we would gather and celebrate the distinctly Greek holidays. Those days would be filled with food, family, and togetherness at pappou and yiayia's house. The salad served would always be yiayia's tart, vinegar-rich recipe. As a mostly herbivorous child, teenager, and adult, I ate the tangy mix frequently. My dad is a huge fan of vinegar, too. I've often wondered if it is a Greek trait or if it runs in our family. In ancient Greece and Rome *posca* was the most common drink. It was water with vinegar and/or wine added to sanitize it for drinking. Herbs, spices, and honey were added in different quantities and mixtures at different times in history.

Apple cider vinegar (ACV) has long been a staple in recipes and in home remedies. Some believe it is an age-old secret and a fountain of youth ingredient that you already have in your kitchen. It is known for its efficacy in treating a variety of health concerns. Most famously, it is touted as an antidote to acid reflux and heartburn. It is reported to lower cholesterol. Many people swear by it for assisting them with healthy weight loss. It's also used to control insulin and blood sugar. It's helpful in treating infections and balancing the body's pH and so much more.

Many people report their grandmothers treating heartburn with a teaspoon of ACV. Some people remember their mothers encouraging them to drink some ACV mixed with water every night before bed for their health.

ACV is a nonalcoholic spirit. It's made from apples that are fermented by living organisms. In historical mystery schools in Greece and the Middle East, fermentation was considered an alchemical process. If you look at it from a mystical perspective, fermentation is a magical, chemical reaction that illustrates the wonder of our natural world. Living organisms change one substance into another.

Apples have a long historical pedigree as a natural cure. Apples are known in many mystical traditions as a symbol of feminine divinity. Mesopotamian mythology talks about a love and fertility goddess named Astarte, whose symbol was the apple.

When you cut an apple in half horizontally, the seeds form the shape of a five-pointed star. You might remember making apple stamps as a child because of this beautiful design contained within the fruit. Astarte was known as the morning star and was a mythological precursor to the Greek goddess Aphrodite and the Roman goddess Venus. Astarte's symbol was considered to be the apple because she was reported to be from the stars.

The seemingly ordinary apple has a rich history. Read on to discover how the effervescent fermentation process undertaken by apples to create ACV can improve our health

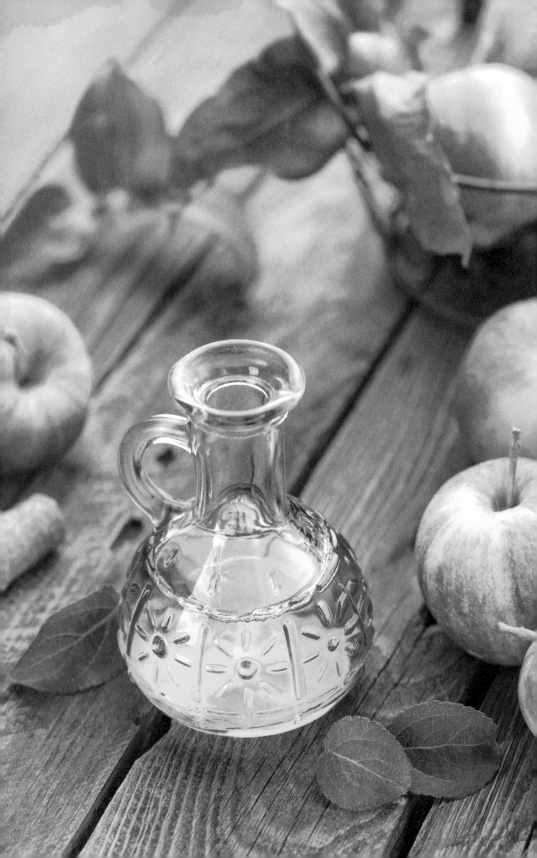

Chapter 1

The History of Apple Cider Vinegar

Vinegar has been around since 5000 BCE. During that time, the Babylonian civilization used it as food and as a preserving or pickling agent. This practice then traveled to other ancient cultures. Vinegar residues have been found in ancient Egyptian urns traced to 3000 BCE.

Legend has it that around 40 BCE, Cleopatra, the beautiful queen of Egypt, won a bet with her lover Mark Antony. After a lavish meal, she supposedly dissolved a priceless pearl in vinegar and then offered it to Antony, to show just how much wealth she had at her fingertips.

In China, references to vinegar in historical texts date back to 1200 BCE. In 10th-century China, Sun Tzu, the creator of forensic medicine, promoted washing one's hands with sulfur and vinegar when working on autopsies, in order to avoid infection.

Around 1000 BCE, in the area that would later become Rome, a variety of vinegars were made from wine, dates, figs, and other fruits. The Romans loved to dip their bread into the vinegar and eat it, along with a sumptuous platter of olives, cheese, and grapes, all of which was accompanied by their delicious wines.

Vinegar is mentioned throughout the Hebrew and Christian Bibles. It was used as everything from a food flavoring to medicine to an energizing drink. The Gospels recount how, as Jesus hung from the cross, a Roman soldier held a sponge soaked in vinegar to his dry lips to help ease his thirst. This was a compassionate gesture, since many Romans drank vinegar mixed with water as a beverage. In the Book of Ruth, after working hard gathering barley in the fields, Ruth was invited to share a meal of bread dipped in vinegar.

The first reference to the medicinal qualities of vinegar was recorded around 400 BCE by the Greek physician Hippocrates, frequently referred to as the father of modern medicine. For coughs and colds, cleaning ulcerations, and the treatment of sores, Hippocrates prescribed ACV mixed with a touch of honey. In the preserved writings from this period that have been ascribed to Hippocrates, he prescribed vinegar for numerous ailments.

In "On the Articulations," which dealt with joint problems, Hippocrates suggested, "If no fever is present, the administration of hellebore [also known as winter rose or Lenten rose], but otherwise it is not to be given, but oxyglyky [a decoction of honeycombs and vinegar] is to be given to drink."

Roman soldiers used to drink a vinegar tonic called *posca* for strength. It was a commonplace drink from 300 to 200 BCE and into the Byzantine period, when it took on the name *phouska*. Both ordinary people and soldiers in the army drank *posca*. It was a beverage looked down upon by the upper classes. This *posca* was made from acetum—a low-quality, sometimes even spoiled, wine or vinegar—as well as herbs, spices, and water. It was actually quite healthy, since it was full of antioxidants and vitamin C and its acidity killed all the bacteria that would have been found in water during premodern times.

ROMAN *POSCA* RECIPE

Serves 4

Just for fun, why not try this adapted *posca* recipe? We can't know exactly how it was made, but based on what we do know, here is a good guess.

    1 cup organic ACV

    ½ cup red wine vinegar

    ½ cup honey

    1 tablespoon crushed coriander seed

Mix all ingredients with 4 cups of water. Boil the mixture so that the honey dissolves. Let it cool to room temperature. Filter out the coriander seeds. Serve in thick glass goblets and enjoy.

The Middle East gave much importance to vinegar. The renowned alchemist Jabir Ibn Hayyan (circa 721–815 CE), who would later be called the father of chemistry, made an extensive study of vinegar and was credited with the discovery of acetic acid, which he obtained through distillation. Islamic alchemists in the eighth century had a more profound knowledge of the chemical properties of vinegar than their European counterparts. Jabir wrote several books that were translated into Latin and became reference works for European alchemists, particularly the *Book of the Composition of Alchemy*.

Another Islamic scientist, Ibn Sina (circa 980–1037 CE), better known in the West as Avicenna, wrote the five-volume encyclopedia *The Canon of Medicine*, in which he mentions the properties and uses of vinegar. According to Avicenna, vinegar is a potent clotting agent that heals burns and skin inflammations, is a good digestive aid , and can be used as an expectorant.

In Europe during the Middle Ages, vinegar had many uses. It was mixed with sand and used to clean and polish chain-mail armor. Parisians used it as a deodorant and a healing tonic, and also believed it preserved youthfulness.

Alchemists would pour it over lead to make a sweet-tasting substance they called sugar of lead, which they added to a harsh cider to sweeten and smooth it out. Unfortunately, because of the very poisonous lead acetate, it caused the early death of many European cider drinkers.

In 1394, a group of French vintners developed what is known as the Orleans method of making vinegar. Oak barrels were used as fermentation tubs and vinegar was expelled from the barrel's base. Roughly 15 percent of the vinegar was left behind, which contained the "mother of vinegar," the concentrated beneficial bacteria hovering on the top. To make a new batch, cider or wine was carefully added to the barrel, which was quick-started by some remaining vinegar intentionally left there. This was called the continuous barrel fermentation method, with which they started producing better supplies of vinegar.

During the Renaissance, Europe's vinegar industry blossomed, and new varieties of flavored vinegar were continually introduced.

In the 17th and 18th centuries, European aristocracy had the custom of holding vinegar-soaked sponges to their noses to ward off the noxious odors of outdoor garbage and raw sewage in cities. They used tiny silver boxes called vinaigrettes, which contained little sponges steeped in vinegar. They could also be stored in compartments inside the heads of walking canes. By the 18th century, there were more than 100 varieties of vinegar infused with herbs, spices, fruits, and even flowers on the market.

Vinegar was even thought to help with preventing the bubonic plague, which killed tens of millions of people during repeated breakouts that started in the 14th century. At one point during the early 18th century, the plague so devastated some French cities that they had trouble burying all of their dead decently. To help cope with the massive number of infected corpses, the French authorities released condemned convicts from prison to help dig the graves. The story goes that while most of these convicts died, one group of four apparently managed to survive by drinking large amounts of vinegar infused with garlic every day. Hence, the garlic-steeped vinegar sold in stores today is still known as "four thieves vinegar."

Pl. 6.

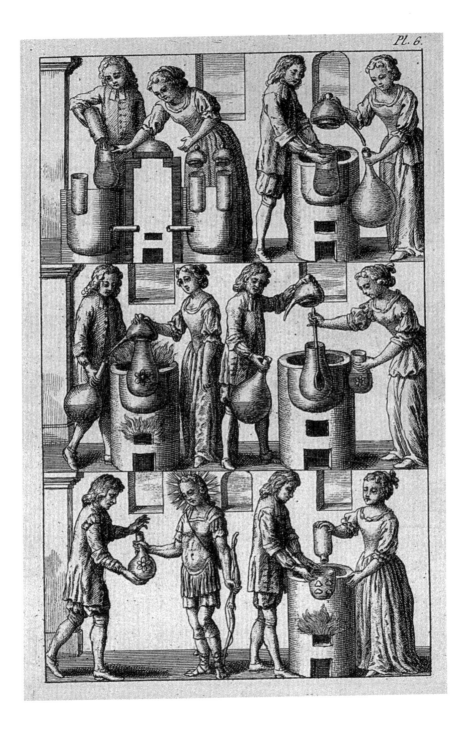

The History of Apple Cider Vinegar

Because of the antiseptic properties of vinegar, it was applied to efficiently disinfect wounds. On his many long sea voyages, Christopher Columbus made sure that his boats were well stocked with barrels of vinegar for this purpose, and also to prevent scurvy in his sailors. Vinegar was still being used to disinfect soldiers' wounds as recently as World War I.

Vinegar has been used for a long time as a folk remedy. It is, in fact, the mainstay of many folk recipes that have been handed down from generation to generation. The main reason it has been used as a remedy is because of its many health-enhancing properties.

It contains a small amount of protein and carbohydrates, plus sodium, potassium, calcium, magnesium, phosphorus, iron, zinc, and chlorine. Long praised for its powerful antioxidants and antiseptic power, it also stimulates circulation, helps detoxify the liver, purifies the blood, cleanses the lymph nodes, and improves immune system response.

WHERE APPLE CIDER VINEGAR BEGAN

Several varieties of smaller wild crabapples are native to North America. But it was the Western European settlers who introduced a more substantial, more useful dessert and cider apple. Most apple trees were propagated by seed, and only some grafted stock was imported from Europe. Only grafted stock produce apples that are the same as the mother tree. Apple trees grown from seed produce fruit that is often different from the mother plant—this is how so many new types of American apples were produced. Wherever American settlers went, they relied on apples, apple cider, and vinegar for food, drink, food preservation, and for medicinal purposes.

In 1623, English clergyman William Blackstone planted some of the first apple trees in Boston. He planted an entire orchard in Rhode Island in 1635 and is credited by many with creating America's first native apple variety, Blaxton's Yellow Sweeting.

As America's settler population increased, more homesteads were built and more apple trees were planted. Ripened apples fed livestock and people. Some of the crop was dried and stored in a cold cellar. Some was made into apple juice by cutting and pressing the apples. This juice fermented into hard cider and was the drink of choice all year for all ages.

Some of this hard apple cider was then allowed to ferment further to produce ACV. This was then used for medicinal purposes, as a condiment, for household cleaning products, and as a preserving liquid for fresh vegetables. By 1775, as many as one-tenth of all New England farms owned and operated cider milling and pressing machinery.

During the early 1800s, John Chapman, also known as Johnny Appleseed, became a folk hero by sharing apple seeds with frontier settlers and starting many nurseries throughout the territories that became the American Midwest. He planted seeds he had bought from cider mills in Pennsylvania. At that time, apples were so integral to American frontier life that the law required each of the settlers to plant 50 apple trees during their first settling year. This ensured that every farm had an apple orchard and a cider press. They produced a refreshing and energizing tonic made from ACV that they would enjoy while doing jobs requiring heavy labor like haying and harvesting. Oftentimes, the vinegar was diluted with fruit juice into a punch-like drink that came to be known as switchel or haymaker's punch.

Because of their bountifulness and utility, apple cider and ACV became a common unit of exchange, especially in rural areas where currency was relatively scarce. Apple cider, in particular, was used as currency to pay for local services, such as those provided by doctors, teachers, and the clergy. It flourished widely. In fact, pioneer pomologist (someone who studies the cultivation of fruit) William Coxe reported that by 1817 in the mid-Atlantic states, apple cider was selling for about $5 per hogshead (about 63 US gallons).

The value of ACV has been heralded in many places all over the world for eons.

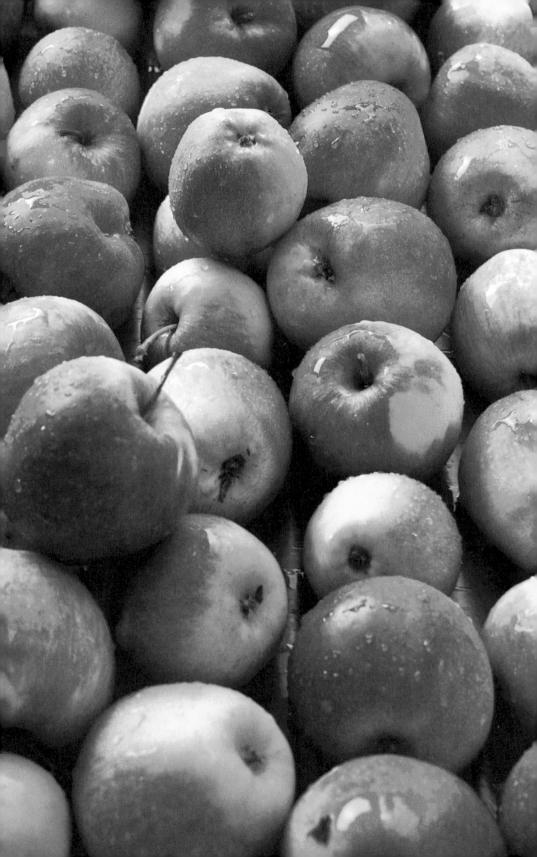

Chapter 2

All About Fermentation

". . . observe the first tiny bubble of fermenting yeast, in which was contained an inevitable, alchemical transformation."

—J. K. Rowling

Apple cider vinegar is arguably the most health-promoting of the vinegars. ACV is high in phosphorus, magnesium, potassium, and calcium. It also acts as a probiotic to help replenish gut flora. Many functional and integrative medicine specialists boast the health-promoting powers of ACV. The secret to its health-promoting power is fermentation.

Fermented foods have become increasingly popular in recent years. We are constantly told about the health benefits of incorporating them into our diets. But what makes these particular foods so special?

As people understand more about how foods work to promote healthier living, we realize that using food to ensure better health is nothing new. The craze for fermented foods has been particularly pronounced recently. But why? Fermentation happens during the chemical breakdown of a substance by bacteria, yeasts, or other microorganisms. But what does that mean?

A further look into the process of fermentation shows that the sugars in fruits are turned into alcohol, and then infused with live organisms that create acetic acid, which is the main compound in vinegar. This vinegar has elements of proteins, enzymes, and healthy bacteria, known as probiotics, that aid in digestion, immunity, and bowel health.

LOWERS BLOOD SUGAR LEVELS AND HELPS FIGHT DIABETES

ACV acts to improve insulin sensitivity, which results in lower blood glucose levels and improves carb breakdown. Diabetes occurs when the body does not respond properly to insulin, which will result in not being able to break down sugars properly. Type 2 diabetes is resistance to the insulin being produced in the body, and the risk of developing it increases with age.

It is possible that ACV can help reduce the effects of type 2 diabetes. As the activity of insulin is stabilized and the blood sugar levels are reduced, a more optimal functioning hormonal balance can be achieved, which reduces the effects of the disease. As the hormones come back into balance, weight loss can occur, which leads to better overall health and more energy.

CAN ACT AS A DISINFECTANT

The powers of bacteria in ACV inside of the body translate outside of the body as well. ACV has been recognized as a treatment for nail fungus, ear infections, warts, and other bacterial ailments. Additionally, ACV works as a surface cleaning agent. ACV is also used as a natural food preservative, as it greatly reduces the spread of bacteria such as *E. coli*.

CAN AID IN LOSING WEIGHT

In addition to its power to lower blood sugar levels, ACV is also known for producing satiety. ACV taken with high-carb meals can increase that full feeling, which leads to an intake of fewer calories. With reduced calorie intake, weight loss can occur over time. But besides that, how does ACV work to promote weight loss?

Protein Utilization

ACV enhances growth hormone, which is essential to digestion. By increasing the acid in the stomach, the growth hormone is stimulated, which increases protein, which in turn helps the growth hormone thrive. This hormone is responsible for the body's metabolism while we are at rest. It's simple: If metabolism is active, it keeps your digestive system going. If it's slower, your body doesn't digest as well.

Digestive Stimulation

Because it aids digestion, ACV helps reduce the time that fats are stored in the digestive tract. Simply put: The faster things can move along, the less chance the fats will be absorbed into the body.

Iron Utilization

Iron acts a fire starter for fuel in the body. Iron carries oxygen through the body, which turns into energy. The better the function of oxygen, the more efficient energy becomes, and the more it works to support weight loss.

CAN TREAT ACID REFLUX AND HEARTBURN

Bacteria living in the gut can cause painful burns in the belly or acid reflux that causes heartburn. Over time, prolonged exposure to and occurrence of acid reflux and heartburn can cause issues with gastrointestinal (GI) tract function, which creates difficulty in digestion. Oftentimes, the overgrowth of the bacteria in the GI tract is due to an imbalance of pH and lack of enzymes and probiotics.

ACV is full of the enzymes and probiotics needed to restore the pH balance in the GI tract, which reduces the amount of acid reflux that causes painful heartburn. With a stronger gut and better digestion, the body can absorb nutrients more efficiently, which will increase energy and overall function.

CAN HELP TREAT THE COMMON COLD

Although the common cold is a virus, it creates harmful bacteria. Because ACV contains plenty of vitamins and acetic acid, it can take charge and kill those nasty bacteria that have built up from the common cold.

BUT WHY IS ACV BENEFICIAL?

Let's start with understanding the gut microbiome, also known as gut flora. The gut microbiome is the complex habitat in which microorganisms live in the digestive tract of mammals. In humans, the gut microbiota contains the highest numbers of bacteria and most species compared to other parts of the human body.

In short, your gut contains a micro city of organisms that work together to keep everything functioning properly. These microorganisms work in your gut to keep diversity, vitality, and variety of the flora.

In order for this to function properly, however, a healthy amount of fermented foods must be included in a diet. Without fermented foods, these microorganisms start to starve and die, which creates a hostile environment in the gut, and bad bacteria start to form. In extreme cases, these bad bacteria thrive and contribute to the perfect environment for cancerous cells in the colon to grow.

ACV creates a defensive barrier against these cancerous cells and keeps the gut microbiome buzzing, functioning, and happy by providing cultures for good bacteria to thrive.

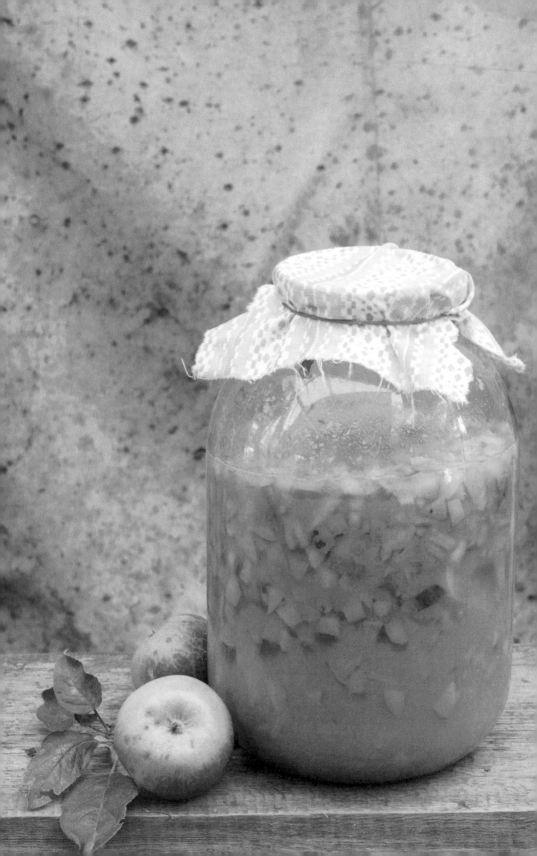

THE PROCESS OF FERMENTATION

ACV is made by crushing apples and squeezing out the liquid. Next, bacteria and yeast are added to the liquid to start the first fermentation process, which is when the sugars are turned into alcohol. In a second fermentation process, the alcohol is converted into vinegar by acetic acid–forming bacteria (acetobacter). Acetic acid gives vinegar its sour taste.

The most important key to a properly fermented ACV is to keep the mother culture intact. The mother is a collection of complex beneficial acids that provide the health-promoting microorganisms and can come in the form of a symbiotic culture of bacteria and yeast, or SCOBY.

In a properly fermented product, you will need to create a SCOBY, which is necessary as it's a home for yeast and good bacteria, but the SCOBY also seals off the fermenting cider from the air and protects it from undesirable outside bacteria while it's fermenting.

Be warned: SCOBY is rather unsightly. It looks a bit like a mushroom or fungi, but that is all looks. The uglier it is, the healthier the SCOBY is.

WAYS TO GET SCOBY-INFUSED ACV

You can get a store-bought ACV with the mother intact. If the ACV you are considering using is murky, brownish, and has a cobweb-like residue in it, you have found a good-quality fermented product. The cobweb-like substance is actually live yeast and bacteria, the elements that promote a healthy gut.

MAKE YOUR OWN ACV

Try making your own ACV with a SCOBY. The process can be long, but it's not hard. A little patience and time will go a long way.

STEP 1: Gather your materials. You'll need a sterilized work area, preferably organic apples, raw sugar, filtered water, and a sterilized, wide-mouth jar.

STEP 2: Wash and chop the apples into medium-sized pieces, and place them in the clean, rinsed, and sterilized wide-mouth jar.

STEP 3: Mix 1 tablespoon of raw sugar with 1 cup of filtered water, and pour on top of the apples.

STEP 4: Cover the jar with a paper coffee filter, and secure tightly with a rubber band. This is essential to allow the mixture to breathe but also keep the bad bacteria away.

STEP 5: Ferment the mixture in a warm spot, around 70°F, out of direct sunlight.

STEP 6: After 7 days, check to see if a baby SCOBY has developed across the surface of the liquid. (If after 3 weeks nothing has happened, start the process over.)

STEP 7: After 2–3 weeks, strain out the liquid and discard the apple pieces.

STEP 8: Return the liquid to the same jar, cover with the same filter, and return it to the same place out of direct sunlight, for an additional 4–6 weeks. Stir the liquid every few days with a wooden or plastic spoon.

STEP 9: After 4–6 weeks, your ACV should be ready to go.

ACV has numerous health-promoting powers for longevity and sustainable quality of life. It's one of nature's oldest treats, and it's something you can make in the comfort of your own home. Thousands of years can't be wrong.

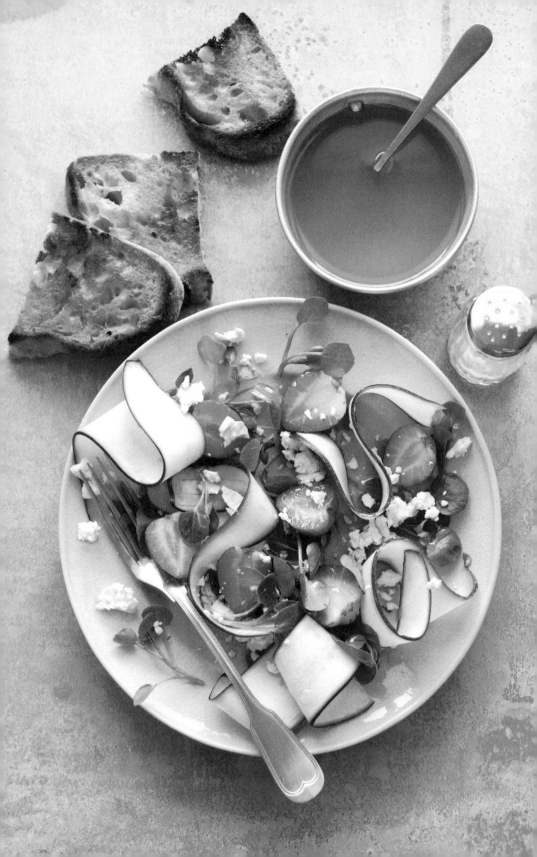

Chapter 3

The Body's Acid and Alkaline Balance

You're reading this because you want to improve your health and have more vitality. So far, you've done your part—you exercise, try to eat a varied diet with plenty of fruit and vegetables, and avoid sweets. You drink green tea and have a serving of protein with each meal. Basically, you're doing everything right. Why are you still battling with low energy?

YOUR ACID-ALKALINE BALANCE

The answer may be simple and something that is often overlooked: Your acid-alkaline balance might be out of whack. The body needs to maintain a slightly alkaline pH of around 7.4 in order to maintain good health. Readings above this level are considered alkaline. Readings that fall below this level are considered acidic.

WHY IS IT HEALTHIER TO BE MORE ALKALINE?

What you eat drastically affects your body's acidity levels. While the occasional imbalance will not cause major problems, a consistently imbalanced pH will. This is one area where you don't want to be an overachiever, especially when it comes to extra acidity.

If you consume a diet that is high in acid-forming foods such as meat, sugar, and dairy, your body will get to a point where it is not able to neutralize all the acid. This, in turn, can cause the following issues.

ACCELERATED AGING: Do you want to look young for as long as possible? Then put that red meat down and step away slowly. When the cells in your body are exposed to extra acidity over the long term, they start to lose structural integrity. The cells are not able to function as well as they should. Add in the damage from pollution and stress, and you have a perfect storm for premature aging.

IMPAIRED BRAIN FUNCTION: Have you been battling to remember things or having trouble focusing? It could be a problem with overacidity. Too much acidity in your system makes it harder for neurons to form as they should. That means that your brain will not be firing on all cylinders, and you won't be able to think as clearly.

DEMINERALIZATION: In order to neutralize excess acids in the body, your system needs to draw on its store of alkaline minerals. These minerals include potassium, magnesium, and calcium. They are stored throughout the body, and concentrated in the bones and teeth. Again, having excess acidity once in a while is not a problem, but when the levels of acidity become consistently raised, the body draws on more of its internal stores, leading to demineralization. If you don't replenish these stores, your bones and teeth become weaker and your risk of developing osteoporosis increases. Demineralization can also result in dry skin that cracks easily, thinning and fragile hair, gum disease, and poor nail health.

FATIGUE: This is a particularly debilitating symptom that most people with an overacidic system battle with. The more acidity in the body increases, the more fatigue you can expect to experience. This is as a result of a general increase in inflammation and a general decrease in the efficiency of the cells in the body. The whole process of energy production slows down dramatically as a result. The amount of oxygen carried to the cells also decreases, which makes it a lot harder for your body to repair itself. The body becomes more prone to attacks from disease and microorganisms such as fungi and yeasts. This can affect the balance of electrolytes in the system, which further disturbs the energy production process.

DISRUPTED ENZYME ACTIVITY: Your body relies on enzymes for just about every one of its functions, from breathing to the absorption of vitamins and minerals to hormonal activity. Extreme acidity in the body can disrupt the action of the enzymes.

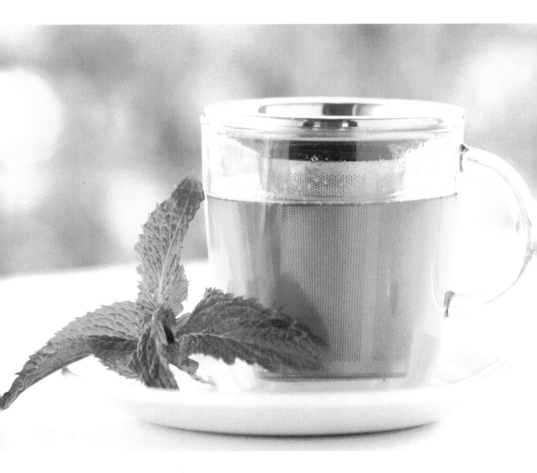

INFLAMMATION AND ORGAN DAMAGE: When there is too much acid in the body on a consistent basis, the tissues become inflamed. Over time, the organs also start to show signs of damage in that they harden and develop lesions. The skin and kidneys are the two organs that are first affected, as their job is to get rid of the excess acid. Eczema, blotchy skin, and hives are all symptoms of having too much acidity in the blood. Excess acidity can also cause the urinary tract to become inflamed, sometimes leading to painful urination and increasing your chances of developing a urinary tract infection.

MORE PRONE TO INFECTION: Excess acidity in the system makes it more vulnerable to infection because excess acidity will impair the proper functioning of the immune system. The number of white blood cells are reduced, and the cells themselves are not as well formed. The immune system becomes unable to perform at full capacity.

CONDITIONS IMPROVE FOR HARMFUL MICROORGANISMS: When the body is in good health and in a balanced state of acidity, it is harder for microorganisms of any sort to get a foothold. On the other hand, when the body is too acidic, the harmful microorganisms are able to flourish because there is less oxygen available in the blood in general. This leads to our own beneficial bacteria becoming overwhelmed.

On the whole, it is far healthier to have a blood pH balance that is slightly more alkaline in nature. Knowing that, you may be tempted to cut out all acid-forming foods altogether. That would be a serious error, though. You will also get sick if your body's alkalinity is too high for an extended period of time.

YOU NEED SOME ACIDITY

The pH in our bodies can change quite a lot from one area to the other. Take the stomach, for example, where the pH is between 1.35 and 3.5. This is as it should be—the stomach needs the additional acidity in order to digest the food that we eat.

The acidity here performs another function as well, though—it kills off microbial organisms that could make us very ill if left unchecked.

Your skin is another area of your body that is quite acidic—between 4 and 6.5. In the morning, the pH of your urine should be between 6.5 and 7.5. You can test your body's acid and alkaline balance using pH test strips.

GETTING THE BALANCE RIGHT

There are people who will tell you that being a vegan is the only way to get the full benefit of an alkaline-based diet. The truth is that while red meat and some forms of dairy form acid in the body, you don't have to go to the extreme of never eating them again.

As always, moderation is the key here. You can still eat meat, nuts, and other acid-causing foods as long as you limit the quantities. As long as about 70–80 percent of your diet is alkaline-forming, you will still be able to indulge in your favorites.

As you would expect, highly processed foods and those with a lot of sugar in them should be limited to very occasional treats, as these are highly acid-forming and also lacking in nutrients. Fresh fruits and vegetables are the foods you want to try to eat the most. You also need to include some fermented foods such as apple cider vinegar, sauerkraut, and miso as well.

Let's break it down so you can see what you should be eating more of, and what foods to avoid, at a glance.

Alkaline-Forming Foods: 70–80 Percent of Your Diet	Neutral Foods: Eat in Moderation	Somewhat Acid-Forming Foods: Eat in Moderation	Acid-Forming Foods: 20–30 Percent of Your Diet
Most fresh vegetables	Pumpkin seeds	Sourdough bread	Meat
Fruit	Yogurt	Spelt	Shellfish
Legumes	Tofu	Brown rice	Sausages
Fruit syrups	Soy milk	Pistachios	Egg whites
Honey	Amaranth	Cashews	Refined flour
Most seeds	Buckwheat	Sesame seeds	Aged cheese
Sprouts	Millet	Hazelnuts	Tea and coffee
Herbs and spices	Quinoa	Almonds	Candy
Olives	Butter	Cottage cheese	Chocolate
Capers	Egg yolks	Fresh cheese	Fish
Sauerkraut	Sunflower seeds	Dry wine	Corn
Yeast		Beer	Rice
Herbal tea		Milk	Pasta
Soy sauce			Alcohol
Apple cider vinegar			Fizzy drinks
			Light breads
			Refined sugar

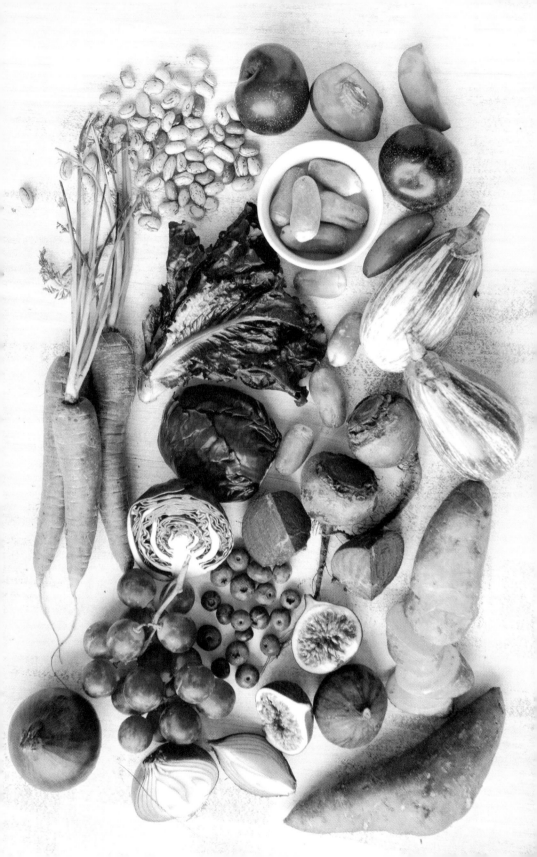

THE BENEFITS OF FERMENTED FOODS

It might surprise you to find that ACV and soy sauce are on the list of alkaline-forming foods. After all, vinegar is acidic, isn't it? This is true.

But there are certain fermented foods, such as kimchi, ACV, and miso that are especially valuable when it comes to your overall health. They act as prebiotics that feed beneficial gut bacteria. This helps to keep your entire system in balance.

And, strangely enough, when they are metabolized by the body, they become alkaline. But no, you can't down a bottle of normal vinegar if you want to alkalinize your system

THE PROPERTIES OF ACV

ACV with the mother is different from normal vinegar. Naturally made ACV is as close as you can come to a perfect food. Since the storied physician Hippocrates used it to treat a variety of ailments, ACV has been known as a powerful healing tonic that has a natural antiseptic and antibiotic effect. It is effective against mold, bacteria, and viruses.

Because it has been fermented, ACV contains a large quantity of acetic acid. This is believed to be one reason that it is so healthy for you. When acetic acid is metabolized, it has an alkalizing effect and can help in reducing acidity in the system. To reap its full benefits, including all the nutrients and phytochemicals present in ACV, it must have the mother culture present in the mixture.

All this means is that your vinegar will be a little cloudy and you may see strands of the yeast used to ferment the apple juice in it. The yeast is beneficial for your system and acts as a prebiotic, helping the healthy bacteria in your system get the upper hand again.

In addition, the acetic acid in the ACV helps to increase the absorption of minerals from the food you eat. Add in the extra enzymes that form during the fermentation process and you have a superfood for your digestive tract. These enzymes help your digestion and cellular function to be more efficient.

TAKING ACV

To use ACV as an alkalizing digestive tonic, you need to take 1 tablespoon of the vinegar diluted in a glass of warm water 15 minutes before each meal. Don't even think of taking it undiluted—you risk damaging your teeth and even burning your esophagus.

Later in the book we will learn a variety of ways to consume ACV and sample an array of delicious recipes.

EATING MORE ALKALINE-FORMING FOODS

Fortunately, you won't have to completely give up all the foods that you love in order to increase your body's alkalinity. You just need to ensure that you eat them in moderation. Commit to cutting acid-forming foods down to less than 40 percent of your diet at most for the next 2 weeks and see how you feel at the end of that. It will be tough in the beginning as your body starts to detoxify itself. Once it begins to get back into balance, however, you'll never want to go back.

Many people feel and look younger on an alkaline-based diet, not to mention having more energy and zest for life. You'll want to eat right and exercise, and you'll have the energy to prepare healthy meals. You'll be able to get on that bike and ride like the wind, even after a long day at work.

Are you ready to get healthy? Are you ready to start getting the most out of life? Getting your body's pH back into balance is the best way to do this, and it doesn't require a bunch of special equipment or expensive supplements.

All you need to do is to review the way you eat—and with a little bit of extra effort, you will receive enormous benefits.

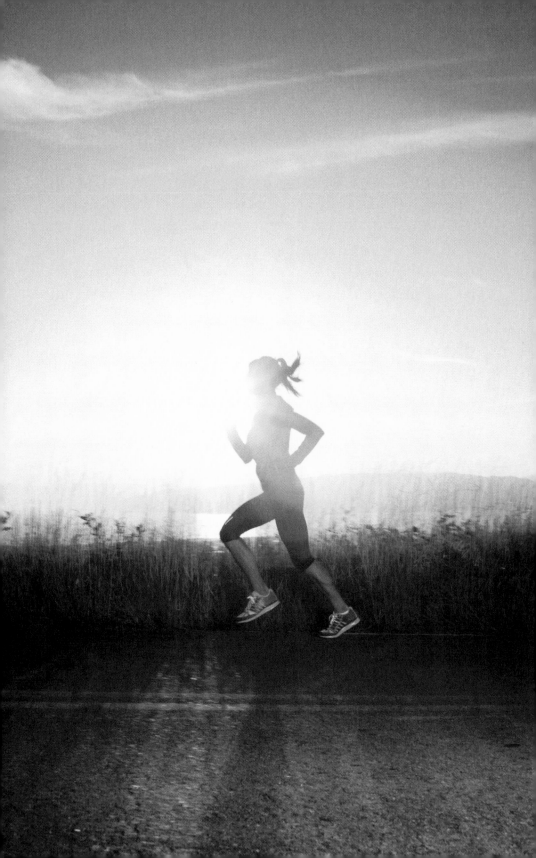

Chapter 4

Apple Cider Vinegar Detoxes and Healthy Weight

"A culture fixated on female thinness is not an obsession about female beauty, but an obsession about female obedience. Dieting is the most potent political sedative in women's history; a quietly mad population is a tractable one."

—Naomi Wolf

In this book, when we talk about healthy weight, we mean what is individually healthy for you. I believe the cultural fixation on people losing weight for health is another form of weight-based prejudice. Fat people are not intrinsically unhealthy. In fact, many are very healthy. They are just shaped differently and look different than what the current media machine (which is designed to sell us things by making us feel we are not good enough without them) shows us we are supposed to look like. What we're talking about in this book is living a lifestyle that enhances your health. Specifically, we are discussing the ways that ACV can help you accomplish this.

I am not telling you that you need to lose weight. I'm telling you to love and care for your body. I'm calling on you to treat your body with the utmost gentleness and regard and put fuel into your body that will help it function optimally. I'm asking you to respect your body and its incredible self-healing and self-regulating capabilities by simply giving it the best possible care.

For some people, detoxifying the body using the natural wonder that is ACV will be very helpful. Our modern lifestyle bombards us with chemicals not only in our foods and drinks but in our environment and in the clothes we wear, the beauty products we use, and the car exhaust we breathe every day. Some of those toxins get stored in the body. Guess where they get stored the most? The areas where there are more concentrated fat cells. Our body wants to encase the toxins in a layer of lipid or fat to encapsulate it so they don't disturb our system.

Because of this, some people who feel like they are not at their optimum weight and want to lose some pounds have a hard time doing so because these fat or lipid layers are housing the toxins that the body is trying to keep out of our primary systems, such as the circulatory and respiratory systems. Detoxifying our body and removing its toxic chemical load in a gentle, manageable manner is one way that we can give our body more resources to process the toxins stored in our fat cells. So, in a roundabout way, detoxification does help us with weight loss if that is the goal that is healthiest for you.

The number one thing you absolutely must do is flush the toxins out. Be certain to drink half of your body weight in ounces of pure, clean water every day. This is a great guideline to begin with. Drinking that much water each day is the ultimate detoxification plan. But when adding in regular doses of ACV for further detoxification, you really need to be flushing out anything that's released so it doesn't sit in the body and get reabsorbed into other areas. So, the more you are detoxing, the more water you need to consume.

For example, if you weigh 160 pounds, then you should be drinking 80 ounces or more of water per day. My acupuncturist and friend Annaliese Klein recommends that you measure this water out in the morning so you are able to see that you have consumed that quantity by the end of the day.

Everywhere you turn, there's another ad for a weight-loss supplement. Drugstore shelves are stocked full of them. They come in various forms: herbal, synthetic, liquids, pills, and powders. But most people don't take the time to discover what's truly in these products and how they might affect the body. In fact, manufacturers aren't required to list all the ingredients of many dietary supplements for those consumers who want to know. Many users of supplements are just looking for a quick fix, which is a complete myth. There is no magic supplement for weight loss. In their quest to shed a few pounds overnight, they're missing the fact that many of these products contain dangerous substances that do more harm than good. In fact, a 2013 study by the Food and Drug Administration found amphetamine-like compounds in several popular supplements. The average person wouldn't knowingly put that in their body.

ACV is a helpful tool in maintaining optimum health. It is best used consistently over time. That is when you will see the most benefit.

Not only are these supplements potentially dangerous, but they're expensive. You could spend thousands of dollars a year on diet pills alone. But supplements aren't the only culprit in terms of cost and toxicity. Some dieting programs are based on people buying prepackaged meals, which are often full of processed foods and artificial sweeteners and colors and preservatives. This route to weight loss can also be a drain on your wallet, with one popular program costing on average $2,500 a year.

Despite all the hyped diet pills and programs, there are still real benefits to optimizing your body weight for health. Remember, healthy body weight is different for everyone. We have numerous genetic and ancestral codes that

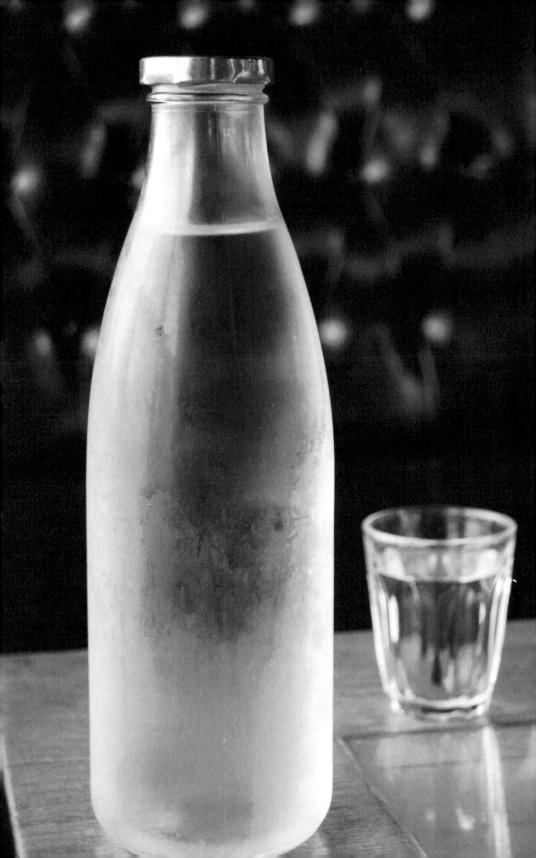

dictate what our bodies should look like and how they should optimally feel. Here are just a few ways that finding your own unique healthy body weight can improve overall health:

* Decreased symptoms of high blood pressure and diabetes

* Increased sex drive

* More energy

* Better sleep

* Improved memory

* Lowered cancer risk

Recently, detox diets like the master cleanse and the grapefruit diet have become all the rage among celebrities and the general public. Some of these remain controversial and potentially harmful for people with certain conditions. The real benefit of detoxification regimens lies in their focus on all-natural foods. Combining a detox regimen with a weight management program not only can help you reach and maintain a healthy weight, but can also cleanse your body of all the gunk that can make you feel terrible. It's hard to exercise and get motivated to prepare healthy meals when you're not feeling your best. What foods can you add to your diet to help you both lose weight and detoxify your body?

Of the many whole food choices out there, ACV is one of the cheapest and most natural food sources to incorporate into a detoxification weight management program. But before we get into the detoxification benefits of ACV, let's dive into why we should worry about toxins in the first place.

TOXINS AND WHERE THEY HIDE

All day long, we are exposed to various chemical compounds. Our body's detox systems are located in the liver, intestines, kidneys, lymph nodes, lungs, and skin. They filter out most of the water-soluble toxins we encounter. However, some of these substances aren't water-soluble and don't get naturally flushed out. Like that houseguest who just won't leave, toxins like to settle in our bodies, particularly in our fat cells. Since they are fat-soluble, they naturally accumulate there. While fat can lock these toxins away where they won't do much damage, the problem arises when we accumulate too much fat in the wrong places, especially around our bellies and around our organs (visceral fat). Toxins stored in this visceral fat can damage our organs and glands, causing them to malfunction. This toxic buildup can lead to several conditions. For example, damage to the pancreas can cause diabetes.

Some common fat-soluble toxins are mercury, PCBs (polychlorinated biphenyls), solvents (such as gasoline, benzene, and xylene), dioxins, many pesticides, many preservatives, many food additives, and toxins from plastic containers.

Toxins aren't just found in our fat cells. They can hang out in other places, like our blood. Those are water-soluble toxins and can usually be filtered out by our liver and kidneys within a couple of hours. The problem comes from our constant exposure. When toxin-laden blood courses through the major systems of the body over long periods of time, it can disrupt hormonal function and damage organs.

Some common water-soluble chemicals are heavy metals (such as lead, thallium, cadmium, and arsenic), chlorinated pesticides, and BPA (bisphenol A).

Other toxins that can damage the body include air pollutants, preservatives, artificial sweeteners, alcohol, and cigarette smoke.

KICKING TOXINS OUT, AKA DETOX

Detoxification (detox) is simply removing toxins that our body can't remove by itself. It sounds daunting, but it really isn't. Remember, your body doesn't actually want to be poisoned.

Benefits of detoxing:

* Improved digestion

* Decreased bloating, gas, constipation, and indigestion

* Deeper and more relaxed breathing

* Decrease in allergic responses to food

* Increased energy

* Weight loss

Think about that last point. Since we tend to store toxins in our visceral fat, a good weight management regimen rids our bodies of this fat and the toxins stored within. Effective detoxification can kick this process into high gear. Along with whole, unprocessed foods, one of the simplest items in your weight management/detox arsenal is ACV.

THE DOUBLE AGENT: ACV

ACV is a jack-of-all-trades when it comes to health benefits, including weight management. But it also works as a detox agent. When both roles work in conjunction, it's a win-win for reaching a healthy weight while flushing out the stuff that kept you from losing weight in the first place. Many studies have shown that ACV can support healthy weight loss.

ACV acts as an appetite suppressant by making you feel full sooner, controls blood sugar levels to combat cravings, prevents fat accumulation by stimulating the metabolism, could help insulin secretion and storage, and detoxifies with insoluble fiber, malic acid, vitamins, minerals, and enzymes.

How do you get ACV to work for you as a weight management and detox agent? First, you must get the right kind. Brand names aren't important, but still, not every ACV is equal. Always look for raw, unprocessed ACV. It contains the cloudy residue known as mother, which packs a lot of ACV's nutritional punch. Also, make a point of seeking out organic ACV. You don't want to buy a bottle of ACV that's been made from apples treated with pesticides. That would defeat the purpose.

> **PLEASE REMEMBER:** Drinking undiluted ACV can erode the tooth enamel. Follow the recommended doses in the recipes for best and safe results.

To activate ACV's weight management and detox power, you just need to incorporate it into your diet. Simply drink 1 tablespoon mixed with a glass of lukewarm water 15 minutes before meals. Then maintain a healthy diet with whole, unprocessed, organic foods. Get plenty of exercise and enough sleep. Drink lots of water. You can also use an infrared sauna to detoxify your body. Try to avoid toxins like cigarettes, alcohol, and plastics. Use natural cleaning and beauty products. Remember, ACV is not a magic weight loss or detox drug. It won't work overnight. Use it daily along with your healthy diet and exercise regimen, and you'll see the results within weeks. Make your ACV intake more interesting with a few simple recipes to spruce up your diet.

Incorporate ACV into your daily routine through substitution. Replace red or white wine vinegar in recipes with ACV. Use it to make salad dressings and in your cooking.

You do not need to try all these recipes in one day. Try one to three per day and find the ones you like best. Try to make a little ACV a daily habit in your healthy lifestyle.

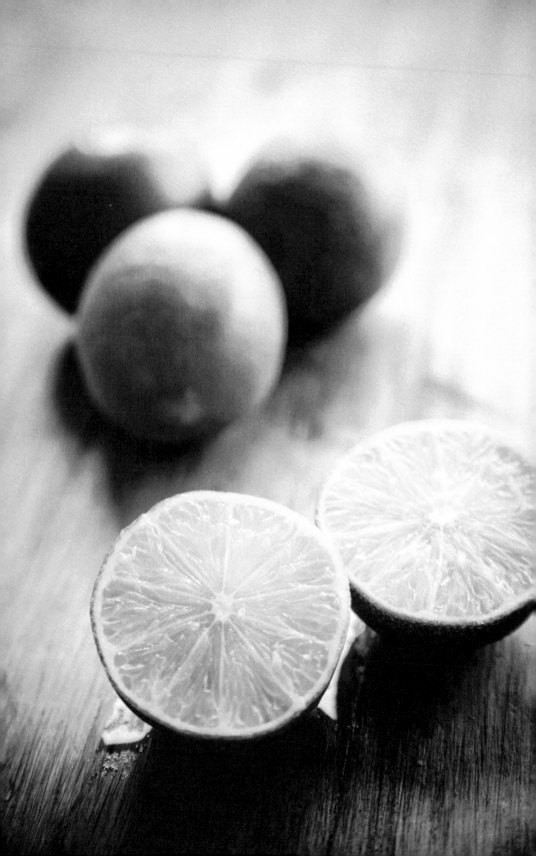

SEASONS

When the seasons change, our bodies respond to the natural cycles of nature. As a result, each change of season offers a beautiful opportunity to cleanse. Detoxification is best done gently. And when a change of season occurs, it's a lovely time to do a very gentle, nurturing, cleansing for body, mind, heart, and spirit.

Spring

When spring dawns, she brings new light and life to the world in every way. This is a lovely time for starting new things and creating new conditions. It's a lovely time for a light, mild internal cellular rinse. Drink the following mixture in the morning to clear and clean your liver and rev up your cells so they can shed the old and welcome the new.

SPRING CLEANSING JUICE

Serves 1

> 4 stalks celery
>
> 4 cups spinach
>
> 1 bunch parsley, plus 1 sprig for garnish
>
> ½ lemon
>
> ½ apple, cored (optional to taste)
>
> ¼ teaspoon ACV

Juice all ingredients except the ACV in a motorized juicer of your choice. Add the ACV and gently stir. Garnish with a sprig of parley.

Summer

Summer favors us with long days, sunshine, and warmth. It is a time when we detox naturally through sweating so we want to support that process gently and allow the body to naturally regulate itself. A dash of ACV will keep your body lightly cleansing in the heat.

SUMMER JOY JUICE

Serves 1

4 cups cubed watermelon

1 lime

1 bunch mint, plus 1 sprig for garnish

1 cucumber (optional—omit if you have seasonal allergies because cucumber can promote histamine production in some people)

¼ teaspoon ACV

Juice all ingredients except the ACV in a motorized juicer of your choice. Add the ACV and gently stir. Garnish with a sprig of mint.

Autumn

Autumn heralds a plentiful harvest and a slight turn inward. When we're in seasonal balance we may reflect in autumn on the excitement of summer and reap the gifts of self-reflection. It is a time when the body wants to stock up on nutrients and vitamins to prepare for the winter ahead. A bit of ACV will keep all the cells of the body from becoming sluggish as we slow down a bit.

FORTIFYING AUTUMN JUICE

Serves 1

1 carrot

3 beets, peeled and cubed

1 bunch kale

½-inch piece ginger, peeled

¼-inch piece turmeric, peeled

1 persimmon, peeled

2 drops ACV

Juice all ingredients except the ACV in a motorized juicer of your choice. Add the ACV and gently stir.

Winter

As it gets cold, we are naturally called to go deeper within the self. Winter is a time for inner alchemy and transformation. It is a time to access our deepest wisdom. Our detoxing in winter must be done with the utmost tenderness and the lightest of touches. This warm drink with just a dash of ACV will keep your body feeling nurtured and allow you to cleanse as needed in the most holistic way for you.

WINTER APPLE WARMER

Serves 1

   1 cup apple juice or apple cider

   2 cups water

   1 clove

   1 cinnamon stick

   2-inch piece ginger, chopped (not peeled)

   Peel of one orange

   ¼ teaspoon ACV

Simmer all ingredients, except for the ACV, in a saucepan on low for 30 minutes. Strain out all the solid ingredients. Pour into a mug and stir in the ACV. Serve warm.

SECRET DETOX DRINK

Serves 1

    2 tablespoons ACV

    2 tablespoons lime juice (liver detox agent)

    ½–1 teaspoon ground ginger or a drop of ginger essential oil

    ¼ teaspoon cinnamon or a drop of cinnamon essential oil

    1 dash cayenne pepper (optional)

    1 teaspoon raw honey

Combine all ingredients, and mix into 12–16 ounces of warm water.
Serve warm.

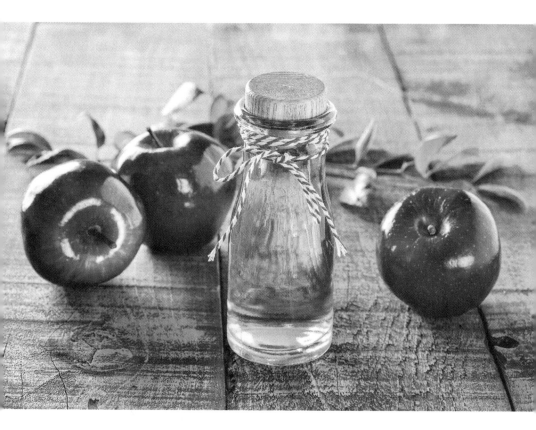

SHAVED GOLDEN BEET, CARROT, AND CABBAGE SALAD

Serves 4

FOR THE DRESSING:

1½ tablespoons ACV

3 tablespoons extra virgin olive oil

2 teaspoons mustard powder

1 teaspoon raw honey

½ teaspoon sea salt

½ teaspoon ground cilantro

Freshly ground black pepper, to taste

FOR THE SHAVED SALAD:

4 small golden beets, peeled

4 medium carrots, peeled and cut in half

1 cup chopped red cabbage

2 tablespoons chopped parsley (diuretic)

Salt and freshly ground black pepper, to taste

Whisk the dressing ingredients in a large bowl. Thinly slice the beets and carrots on a mandoline or in a food processor with a slicing disk. Toss the beets and carrots with the cabbage and dressing until evenly coated. Sprinkle with chopped parsley. Season to taste with salt and freshly ground pepper.

STRAWBERRY-PAPAYA ACV DETOX SMOOTHIE

Serves 1

- 1 organic frozen papaya, peeled and cubed (make sure to use organic because most papayas are heavily sprayed with pesticides)
- ½ cup frozen strawberries
- 1 frozen banana
- ½ cup unsweetened rice milk
- ¼ cup chia seeds
- 1 tablespoon ACV
- 3 ice cubes
- 3 mint leaves

Add all ingredients except the mint to a blender. Blend until smooth. Garnish with mint leaves.

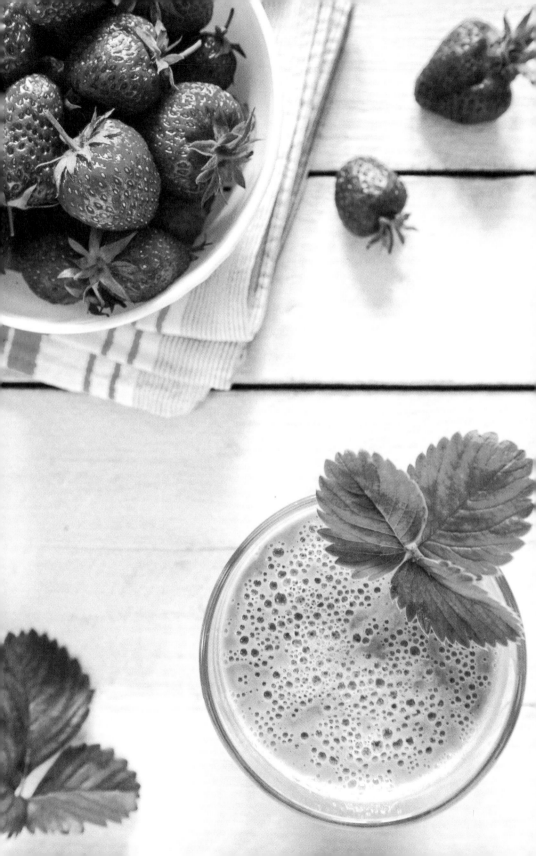

ACV FATOOSH SALAD

Serves 2

   2 cucumbers, sliced

   2 tomatoes, chopped

   4 spring onions, chopped

   ¼ cup diced green olives

   3 tablespoons ACV

   ¼ teaspoon salt

   ¼ teaspoon black pepper

   1 dash of powdered stevia (optional)

Place the cucumbers, tomatoes, onions, and olives in a large bowl. Toss to mix. In a small bowl, combine the ACV with 3 tablespoons of water. Pour over the vegetables. Add the salt, pepper, and optional stevia. Toss well. Store in an airtight container in the refrigerator for up to 4 days.

QUINOA AND ADZUKI BEAN SALAD

Serves 2

1 cup uncooked quinoa (any color), rinsed and drained

1 cup orange juice

¼ cup extra virgin olive oil

2 teaspoons ACV

½ teaspoon honey or agave nectar

2 tablespoons dried cranberries

2 tablespoons chopped walnuts

½ teaspoon salt

Freshly ground black pepper

¼ cup chopped cilantro

1½ cups (or 1 can) cooked adzuki beans, drained and rinsed

½ small red onion, thinly sliced

Place the quinoa, orange juice, and 1 cup of water in a small saucepan. Bring to a boil over medium-high heat. Cover and simmer over low heat for about 15 minutes, or until the liquid is absorbed. Remove from the heat and let stand for 5 minutes. Fluff the quinoa with a fork. Set aside. Combine the remaining ingredients, then stir them into the quinoa. Serve immediately or refrigerate.

CHOCOLATE-ALMOND BUTTER-BANANA MILK SHAKE

Serves 1

½ cup rice milk, almond milk, or soy milk

1 tablespoon almond butter

1 tablespoon ground flaxseed

2 teaspoons raw honey

½ teaspoon pure vanilla extract

½ teaspoon ACV

¼ teaspoon ground nutmeg

1 pinch sea salt

1 ripe banana, peeled and frozen

2 tablespoons raw cocoa or cacao powder

1 teaspoon raw cacao nibs, for garnish (optional)

Place all ingredients, except for the cacao nibs, in a blender. Process until smooth. Pour into a glass. Top with cacao nibs, if desired. Serve immediately.

SALT DETOX BATH RECIPE

Yields 1 bath

¼ cup sea salt or Himalayan salt

¼ cup Epsom salt

¼ cup baking soda

⅓ cup ACV

Favorite essential oils, if desired (rose, chamomile, etc.)

Dissolve the sea salt, Epsom salt, and baking soda in a quart-size jar filled with boiling water. Set aside. Fill your tub with warm or hot water and add the ACV. Pour in the salt mixture. Add about 10 drops of essential oils, if using. Soak in the bath for at least 30 minutes. Note that with any detox bath, you may feel tired or lightheaded when you get out. Note: This bath is best used at bedtime and is great for soothing skin irritations, boosting magnesium levels, and overall detoxing. Make sure to drink lots of water after a detox bath.

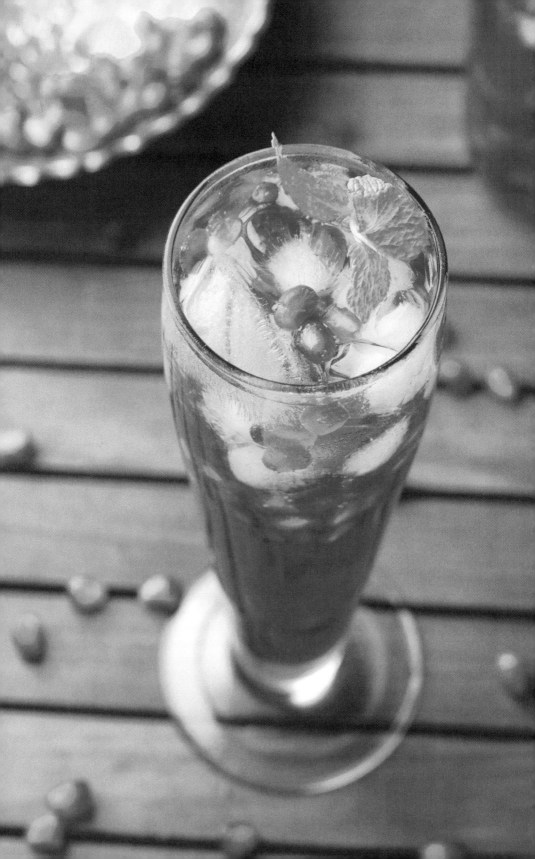

Chapter 5

A Robust Antioxidant and Cancer Preventive

From natural cleaner to sunburn soother, apple cider vinegar has many uses for healthy living. Of those, one of its most important uses may be disease prevention. It's rich in antioxidants, which are known to fight free radicals that can lead to many diseases, including cancer. Since an estimated 40 percent of US citizens are diagnosed with cancer at some point in their lives, it's worth looking at natural sources that could help prevent this dread disease. But what are antioxidants, and how does ACV play a role in cancer prevention?

THE ENEMY: FREE RADICALS

Let's start with the archnemesis of antioxidants: free radicals. These troublesome molecules are natural by-products of our body's own metabolism within each cell. They've lost an electron as part of this process, which makes them electrically charged and unstable. They want that electron back, so they'll pull one from any innocent molecule that may be nearby, thus turning it into a free radical, which then starts a chain reaction that can damage the cell. When free radicals become overabundant, widespread cellular damage, called oxidative stress, can occur. This could affect anything from the cell membrane to the DNA, making the cell die or mutate, which could result in tumor growth.

Studies have linked oxidative stress to many diseases, including macular degeneration, alcoholism, Alzheimer's disease, ulcers, arthritis, and certain cancers. It can also affect our appearance, leading to premature aging. To make matters worse, our lifestyle choices can increase the production of free radicals. Smoking, poor nutrition, drinking alcohol, and chronic stress are some of the main culprits. Free radicals do have a couple of redeeming qualities. When in proper balance, they help cells turn oxygen and nutrients into the chemical energy they need. They also travel through our circulatory system and attack invading bacteria, making them a key player on the immune system team. Free radicals alone aren't responsible for diseases like cancer. The problem comes from having too many of them.

Antioxidants are the solution. These heroes are composed of molecules that inhibit the oxidation of other molecules. They can react with free radicals to take the place of their missing electron, which neutralizes its charge and prevents it from damaging other molecules and harming our cells. But we must include enough of them in our diets to make a difference.

Antioxidants in ACV

There are many types of antioxidants, but they can be divided into three main groups:

1 ENZYMES: produced in the body from proteins and minerals as part of our daily food intake; require co-factors like iron, selenium, copper, zinc, and magnesium.
2 VITAMINS: generally not produced naturally in the body; must come from dietary sources; examples include folic acid, vitamin C, and beta-carotene.
3 PHYTOCHEMICALS: produced naturally by plants to protect them from free radical damage; examples include carotenoids, polyphenols, flavonoids, and allyl sulfides.

Antioxidant supplements can be useful. But the best sources of antioxidants, by far, are whole and minimally processed natural foods. ACV is produced by simple fermentation of yeast in apple juice. It's rich in the phytochemical department, specifically the flavonoids rutin and quercetin, chlorogenic acid, and gallic acid. Research has shown that some phytochemicals could help with cancer prevention by blocking the formation of carcinogens, stopping carcinogens from attacking cells, and helping cells eliminate cancer-causing mutations. How they work on a molecular level to prevent cancer depends on the specific antioxidant and the area of the body it affects. For instance, some phytochemicals, called phytoestrogens, may protect breast cells from cancer by protecting them from estrogen. They bind to estrogen receptors on the cells, but don't facilitate the same level of hormonal activity believed to cause breast cancer.

It's important to note that larger studies of ACV's link to cancer prevention are inconclusive, while smaller studies have shown a link. It is not a patentable substance, and therefore for-profit companies have no incentive to fund studies to determine its efficacy. Even if the cancer-fighting benefits of ACV have not yet been proven, its antioxidants and other health benefits make it worth incorporating into your diet. All you need are a few simple recipes.

ANTIOXIDANT POMEGRANATE DETOX

Serves 2

- ¼ cup organic, not-from-concentrate pomegranate juice (rich in punicalagin)
- 3 tablespoons ACV
- 6–7 drops liquid stevia (more if desired)

Combine all ingredients in a glass with 12–13 ounces of cold filtered water. Stir or shake to mix. Taste and add more stevia if desired. Serve cold, over ice if desired.

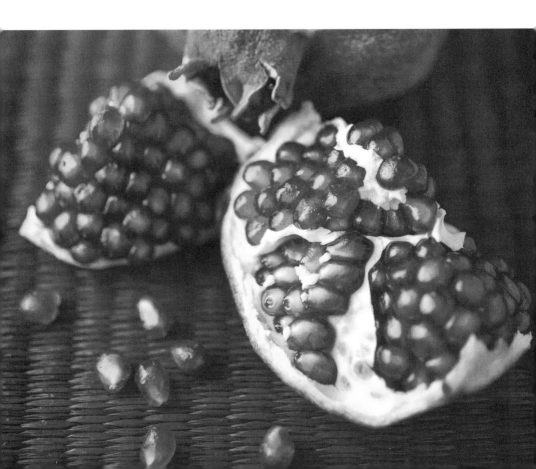

ARUGULA SALAD
WITH ACORN SQUASH

Serves 2

2 tablespoons olive oil (rich in vitamin E)

1½ tablespoons ACV

2 teaspoons lemon juice

1 teaspoon mustard powder

1 teaspoon honey

½ teaspoon dried dill weed

FOR THE SALAD:

3 cups arugula (rich in vitamin A)

1 cup roasted acorn squash, cubed (rich in beta-carotene)

¼ cup goat cheese, crumbled

¼ cup pumpkin seeds (rich in antioxidants)

Combine the vinaigrette ingredients in a jar with a tight-fitting lid, and shake to mix. Set aside. In a large bowl, toss the arugula, squash, and cheese. Add the vinaigrette and toss. Garnish with pumpkin seeds before serving.

TWO-MINUTE HEALTHY KETCHUP

Yields 1¹/₄ cups

> 1 cup tomato paste (rich in lycopene)
>
> ¼ cup maple syrup
>
> 2 tablespoons ACV
>
> 1 teaspoon onion powder
>
> 1 teaspoon dried oregano (rich in polyphenols)
>
> Sea salt (optional)

Combine all ingredients in mixing bowl. Taste and adjust seasonings if necessary.

SALT- AND VINEGAR-ROASTED BUTTERNUT SQUASH

Serves 6

- 2 tablespoons olive oil
- 3 tablespoons ACV, divided
- 4 sprigs fresh rosemary, chopped
- 1 teaspoon salt, divided
- ¼ teaspoon ground black pepper
- 2 pounds butternut squash, peeled and cubed (rich in antioxidants)

Preheat the oven to 400°F. In a large bowl, place the oil, 2 tablespoons of the ACV, the rosemary, ½ teaspoon of the salt, and the pepper. Whisk until well combined. Add the squash. Stir to evenly coat the squash in the vinaigrette. Pour the squash onto a large baking sheet and spread into an even layer. Bake for 25 minutes. Flip the squash pieces with a spatula. Bake for an additional 20 minutes. Loosen the squash from the baking sheet with a spatula. Drizzle with the remaining vinegar and salt. Stir to evenly coat.

ANTIOXIDANT BLAST MUFFINS

Serves 12

½ cup soy milk (rich in phytoestrogens)

1 teaspoon ACV

⅜ cup cornmeal or rice flour

¾ cup whole wheat flour (rich in selenium and vitamin E)

½ teaspoon stevia powder

1 teaspoon cinnamon (rich in many antioxidants)

½ teaspoon nutmeg (rich in many antioxidants)

½ teaspoon cardamom (rich in many antioxidants)

1 teaspoon baking powder

½ teaspoon baking soda

½ teaspoon salt

2 tablespoons ground flaxseeds (rich in vitamin E)

¾ cup cooked quinoa (rich in selenium and vitamin E)

1 tablespoon unsweetened applesauce

¼ cup molasses

¾ cup sweet potato puree (rich in beta-carotene)

2 teaspoons vanilla extract

¼ cup margarine, melted and cooled

¼ cup shelled sunflower seeds or pumpkin seeds (rich in vitamin E)

Preheat the oven to 400°F, and line a 12-muffin pan with paper baking cups. In a small bowl, whisk together the soy milk and ACV and set aside to curdle. In a large bowl, combine the cornmeal, whole wheat flour, stevia, cinnamon, nutmeg, cardamom, baking powder, baking soda, salt, and flaxseeds. Stir to combine. Add the quinoa and stir to distribute it evenly throughout the dry ingredients. In a medium bowl, whisk the applesauce with ¼ cup warm water until frothy. Add the molasses, sweet potato puree, vanilla, margarine, and soy milk/ACV mixture. Mix thoroughly. Add the wet ingredients to the dry ingredients. Stir until just combined. Spoon the batter into the prepared muffin pan. Sprinkle the sunflower seeds on top of the muffins. Bake for 30 minutes or until an inserted toothpick comes out clean.

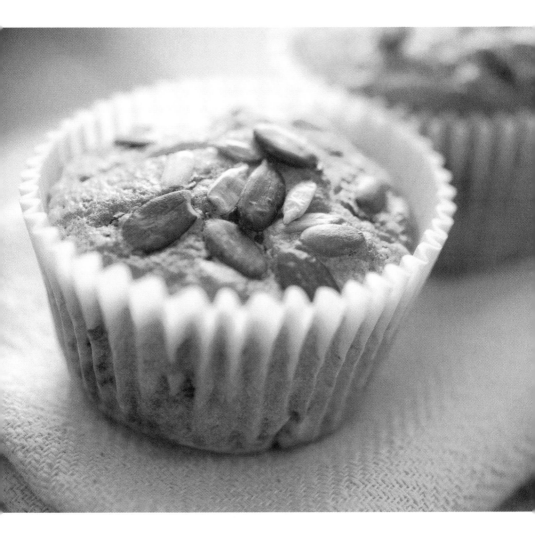

VEGAN "CHEEZE" DIP

Serves 4

2 tablespoons olive oil

½ large yellow onion, finely diced

3 garlic cloves, pressed (rich in allium sulfur compounds)

2 large carrots, minced

1 cup butternut squash, peeled and thinly sliced

2 teaspoons salt, divided

1 teaspoon cumin

½ teaspoon chili powder

¼ teaspoon black pepper

1 cup vegetable stock

1 bunch fresh chives, chopped

1½ cups unsweetened plain almond milk

1 cup cashews, soaked overnight or at least 30 minutes in water, drained (rich in zinc)

¼ cup nutritional yeast

½ cup diced, seeded tomatoes (rich in lycopene)

1 tablespoon ACV

OPTIONAL TOPPINGS:

Pumpkin seeds (rich in antioxidants)

Salted nuts of your choice

Roma tomatoes, chopped (rich in lycopene)

Cilantro (rich in quercetin)

Heat the olive oil in a large saucepan over medium heat. Add the onions and garlic. Sauté until the onions are soft and the garlic is fragrant. Add the carrots and butternut squash. Stir to combine. Add 1 teaspoon of the salt along with the cumin, chili powder, and black pepper. Cook for 2 minutes, then add the vegetable stock. Bring to a simmer, stirring frequently until the vegetables are soft enough to process in a blender. Pour the vegetable mixture into a high-powered blender. Add the chives, almond milk, cashews, nutritional yeast, tomatoes, ACV, and the remaining salt. Blend well, scraping the sides as needed, until the mixture is thick and creamy. Adjust the seasoning as needed. To reheat, gently warm in a pan over low heat to the desired temperature. Serve alongside rice or tortilla chips and garnish with your favorite toppings.

SAGE TURMERIC FIZZ

Serves 1

3 sage leaves (rich in carnosic acid)

1 sprig mint

1 sprig thyme

1 1-inch piece fresh ginger, peeled and chopped

¼ teaspoon turmeric powder (rich in curcumin)

Juice of 1 medium orange (rich in vitamin C)

1 cup club soda (or water)

1 tablespoon ACV

1 tablespoon honey

Muddle the sage, mint, thyme, ginger, and turmeric in a tumbler or glass of your choice. Add the orange juice, club soda, ACV, and honey. Stir until combined. Strain and serve over ice.

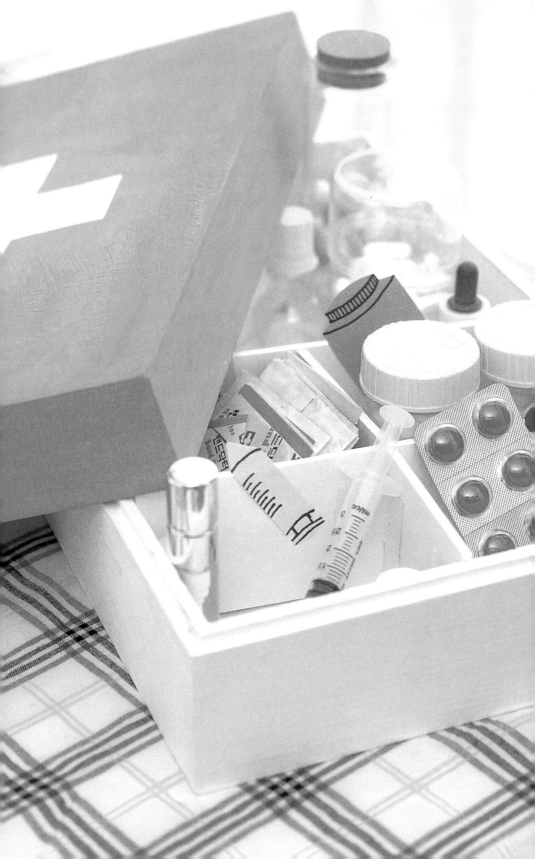

Chapter 6

First Aid and Antibacterial Treatments Using Apple Cider Vinegar

Why is ACV so useful when it comes to overall health? It seems strange that something we eat so little of can have such huge benefits, but to understand why this is, we need to first understand something about the microflora in our own bodies.

A HEALTHY GUT MEANS A HEALTHY LIFE

Would it surprise you to learn that your immune system starts in your digestive tract? In fact, only about 20 percent of your body's immune system exists outside of your digestive tract. Isn't that amazing? It certainly makes you want to think twice about what goes into your gut, doesn't it?

The digestive system is actually part of the neurological system, and that is why it is often referred to as the "second brain." It may seem strange, but many different diseases, from depression to psoriasis, may be the result of the digestive system being unhealthy.

The gut is vital to every system in your body—every system in the body derives its energy from the gut. But we are making it harder for our bodies by loading up on toxins like sugar, processed foods, and the like that actually harm the beneficial bacteria in the gut and make it possible for harmful bacteria to thrive.

This imbalance creates a problem when it comes to effective digestion, and we are not able to get as many nutrients from our foods. The body's systems become far less effective, and chronic inflammation is triggered, setting us up for poor health. Fortunately, you can restore the balance by changing what you eat on a daily basis and including more probiotics.

WHAT ARE PROBIOTICS?

Not all bacteria are bad. In fact, without the beneficial bacteria in our digestive tract, we would not be able to absorb any nutrients or fight off any type of infections. These bacteria are known as probiotics, and while they can be found throughout the whole body, they are concentrated in the gut and the mucous membranes, including the genital tract and the sinuses.

You will find bacteria within your gut and on your skin, warding off disease and keeping you healthy. There are thousands of types of bacteria present in your body right now. That includes good and bad bacteria.

The good bacteria produce vitamins such as K_2 and B_{12}, create enzymes to kill bad bacteria, and compete with bad bacteria and a host of other pathogens for resources.

Should you not have the right number of probiotics, you are at a greater risk of developing skin disorders, digestive upsets, candida, lowered immune function, and autoimmune diseases. You are also likely to have higher levels of inflammation, which comes with its own set of health issues.

Before the advent of refrigeration, this wasn't an issue. We ate tons of fresh fruits and vegetables, grown in nutrient-rich soil. Because we had to get creative about storing foods, we fermented some of them to keep them edible for longer periods.

Now, however, we don't have to worry as much about our food spoiling because it can be refrigerated. Overfarming of the land has led to food being produced that is less nutritious. Also, because we want our food to look perfect, it is often soaked in chlorine or treated with antibiotics to stave off disease and decay.

Just by introducing your body to good probiotic foods, you will strengthen your immune system, enjoy better digestion, get rid of candida, see a reduction in skin issues, and have higher energy levels. You are also likely to be able to lose excess weight and to keep it off.

WHAT IS BAD ABOUT PROBIOTICS?

Most of us are aware that antibiotics can wreak havoc on our system. We know that if we are prescribed an antibiotic, we need to supplement our diets with a probiotic to offset its effects.

What few people know, however, is that they may be ingesting antibiotics in the food that they eat without even realizing it. Non–organically raised livestock are treated with antibiotics as a matter of course. This leaves traces in the meat when the animals are slaughtered.

Another concern is how dangerous sugar is for beneficial gut bacteria. Sugar has minimal nutritional value and is added to most foods simply to improve their flavor. The problem with sugar is it provides the perfect food for bad and pathogenic bacteria like candida to thrive. It leaves the field wide open for dangerous bacteria to gain a firm foothold.

You need to watch out for more than just the sugar in your food. If you are eating highly processed foods, you are also effectively starving your body's good bacteria. Fiber in our diet ensures that we have enough prebiotics to feed the probiotic bacteria. By excluding fiber, we are cutting off another food source for the probiotics.

In addition, the barrage of chemicals and medications that we take on a daily basis are damaging our guts. Even something that seems as innocuous as tap water can be causing a problem—most tap water is fluoridated and chlorinated to sanitize it. These chemicals kill good and bad bacteria alike.

Our stressful lives are not doing us any favors, either. The more stress we are under, the more difficult it is for the probiotics in our systems to thrive. Alcohol is another no-no if you want to restore a healthy balance in your gut.

Your best defense is to start looking at improving your diet overall. To do this, first eat healthy food that has been processed as little as possible. Then, cut out foods that have been processed and start introducing foods that are natural probiotics like kefir and ACV. Also, get enough fiber in your diet to keep the beneficial bacteria happy, and you'll soon start feeling like a new person.

Taking organic ACV on a daily basis will put you ahead of the race. Take our ACV tonic about 15 minutes before eating breakfast, lunch, and supper to get the maximum benefits. It is extremely important to use an unfiltered, organic ACV—the filtered versions have very little of the beneficial bacteria left in them.

Unfiltered ACV looks a little cloudy and may even seem to have strings floating around in it. This is exactly what you want, so don't be put off by the way it looks.

ACV AS AN ANTIBACTERIAL AGENT

It may seem counterintuitive, but ACV is a prebiotic as well. It kills harmful bacteria and supports the growth of the bacteria that are essential for good health. Getting the balance right can be useful when it comes to the prevention and treatment of urinary tract infections and in neutralizing the risk from food-borne illnesses.

It is not just your gut that will benefit, though. New research has shown promising results for your teeth as well. Having the right balance of beneficial bacteria may help to prevent cavities and gum disease. Studies have even linked depression to an imbalance in intestinal flora.

ACV TO DEAL WITH MITES

Our skin has a layer of beneficial bacteria on it. This is a good thing—it helps protect us from disease and parasites. Take demodex mites, for example. These are present on most people, and they feed on dead skin.

Normally, these mites don't cause problems for us, because the beneficial bacteria on the surface of the skin keep them in check. However, if allowed to proliferate, like when our good bacteria are out of balance, they can cause a lot of discomfort.

Demodex mites also carry bacteria on themselves. They can burrow into the skin around the eyes and into the eyelashes, introducing bacteria to these areas that can result in adverse skin reactions and infections. This can result in itchy, fiery inflammations that can be quite unsightly.

Normally, your doctor will prescribe a course of cortisone to help deal with this kind of inflammation. But ACV can provide a natural, more gentle solution. Use the Mite-Busting Remedy on page 83 two to three times a day to get rid of mites.

ACV is an effective treatment because it is antibacterial and so destroys the mite-borne bacteria that cause the inflammation.

It also helps to restore the skin's natural pH balance and acid mantle, making the skin better able to fight off attacks. It mitigates itching associated with the infection, as well.

ACV TO DEAL WITH DANDRUFF

Dandruff can be caused by an overgrowth of skin cells on the scalp. The causes may vary from fungal infections, to a skin condition, to a simple imbalance in the pH level of the skin.

It may surprise you to learn that ACV is a natural treatment that can help you treat dandruff. ACV will help rebalance the skin's pH and make your scalp healthier and so reduce skin problems. If your dandruff is caused by a fungal infection, ACV will help kill off the fungus.

In most cases, all you will need to do is to mix equal parts of ACV and water and massage the mixture into the scalp at least once a day, preferably just after washing your hair.

ACV IN YOUR FIRST AID KIT

ACV has excellent antibacterial properties, but its benefit in your first aid kit go far beyond that, especially when it comes to your skin. It is a natural remedy that reduces inflammation and soothes irritated skin.

It makes for a wonderful treatment for razor burn, for example. Simply mix equal parts of ACV and water and apply to the skin after shaving. The acetic acid in the vinegar will also help soften your skin and prevent ingrown hairs.

ACV and colloidal silver together make an effective treatment for minor wounds and promote the fast healing of the skin. Colloidal silver hydrosol is a clear liquid that is antibacterial, antifungal, antiviral, and anti-inflammatory. It is used topically and internally.

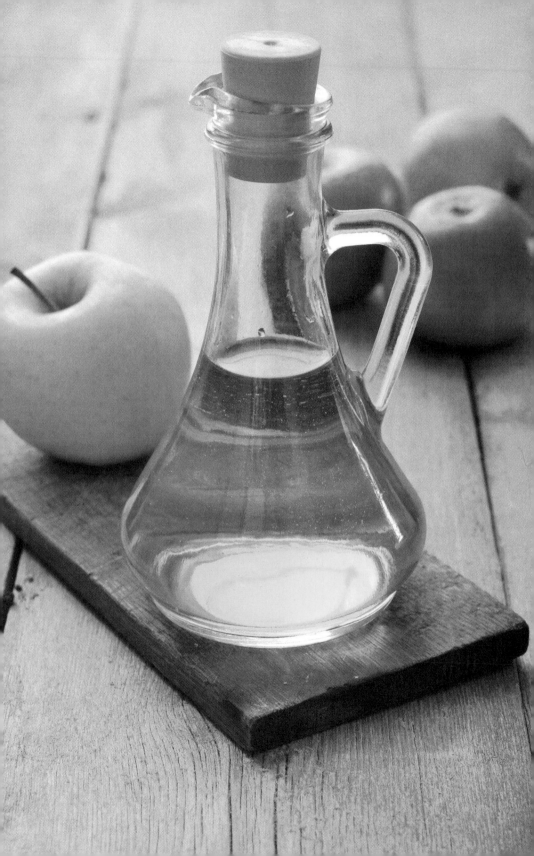

Why Is Organic Better?

BETTER FOR YOUR HEALTH

Corporations are one of the main sources of funding for scientific studies in the United States. Because of this there have been many studies funded by and lobbied for by large agribusinesses, designed to discredit the value of organic farming.

Very few studies exist to prove the value of organic farming because the funding does not exist. There is nothing to patent and so no way to garner profit.

What has been studied is how the nutritional value of fruits and vegetables begins to drop almost immediately after being harvested. One study found that broccoli loses as much as 50 percent of its vitamin C content seven days after being harvested. However, if that broccoli was organically grown, it would likely be consumed more quickly than conventionally grown produce, simply because it wouldn't last as long. It would also be more likely to be consumed locally. Organically grown produce does not have the ability to sit on the shelf for weeks looking perfect because it hasn't been heavily sprayed or genetically modified. Something that is listed as 100 percent organically grown was not sprayed with pesticides and was not genetically modified.

When our food is treated with pesticides designed to kill organisms that would interfere with food production, there is a residue left on them. Those same compounds that can kill bugs and pests can also kill our good bacteria (probiotics). Widespread use of pesticides has been a contributing factor to the dysregulation of our bodily flora and the rise of resulting diseases.

APPLE CIDER VINEGAR TONIC

Serves 1

> 1 tablespoon organic ACV
>
> 1 teaspoon raw honey (optional)

Mix the ACV into 1 cup of water and drink it. Use the raw honey as a chaser to get rid of the taste.

MITE-BUSTING REMEDY

Yields 1 cup

> ¼ cup organic ACV
>
> 3 drops tea tree oil (the number one enemy of demodex mites that are too numerous)

Mix the ACV and tea tree oil into ¾ cup of water. Apply to the affected areas using a cotton ball after cleansing, avoiding the eye area. You can also use this remedy on the rest of your body to help restore the skin's natural pH and deal with other skin ailments caused by mites.

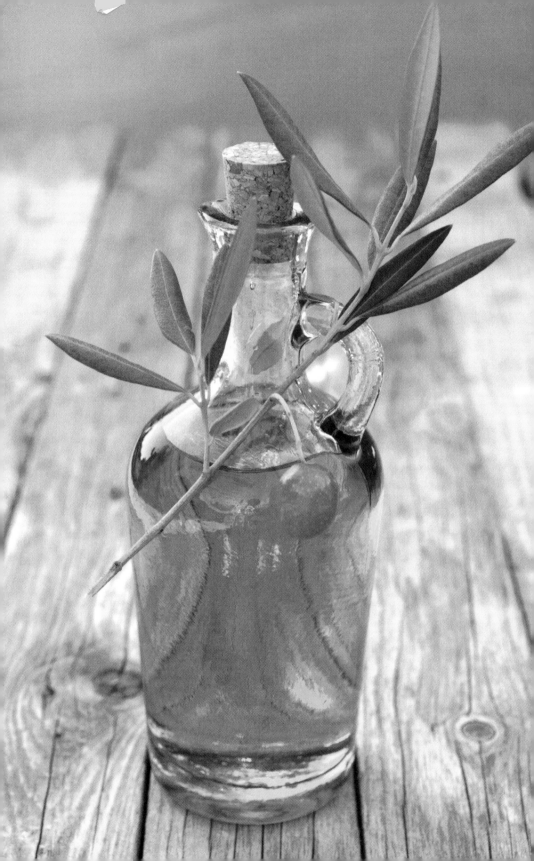

Chapter 7

Improving Nutrient Absorption with Apple Cider Vinegar

Do you sometimes feel like you have a hard lump in your stomach after eating, no matter how much food you eat? Do you experience pain and discomfort after eating? Or perhaps you have a really bloated stomach and gas?

If so, you might have a digestive problem. Now, if this discomfort is happening once in a while, it's not going to be much of a problem. But if it starts to happen often, it can be disconcerting, to say the least. And it really isn't good for you—it's a sign that your digestive system is out of whack.

That is a big problem. An unhappy gut is an unhealthy one, which can upset every other system in your body. Digestive problems can have impacts on your health in ways you would never realize. Did you know, for example, that the levels of microflora in your gut can affect whether or not you feel depressed?

It may seem like a strange connection to make, but the digestive tract forms a large part of your body's neurological system. The term "gut feeling" takes on a whole new meaning, doesn't it?

Add in the fact that most of your body's immune system is in your gut, and the health of your digestive tract becomes a major issue. That beneficial bacteria in the gut are your first line of defense. These microflora are essential for the proper absorption of nutrients from your food and the production of energy and certain vitamins.

It's a system designed to break down our food very efficiently. The problem is, though, that we got far too smart for our own good. We started changing the types of food we eat and modifying food until it is virtually indistinguishable from what it was like in its natural state.

The typical Western diet is loaded with highly processed foods that have been stripped of fiber and most of their nutritive elements. Think about this for a second—why do we have to fortify our food with vitamins? It's because processing strips a lot of the goodness out of them.

Also, processed foods just don't taste that good. To improve their flavor, companies pump in sugar. This wreaks even more havoc on our digestive systems. First, it significantly boosts our blood sugar levels. Second, it starves the good bacteria in our guts and feeds the bad bacteria.

In addition, much of our food is heavily treated with various chemicals, from pesticides to antibiotics, to help protect it from disease and to increase production. The problem with this is that we then consume the residue of these chemicals along with our food, no matter how much we might wash it.

The end result of all this industrialized food is that we end up more vulnerable to bacterial and fungal infections, such as candida, and our health suffers. Faced with a dwindling amount of good bacteria, our digestive tract becomes a lot less efficient when it comes to extracting nutrients from our food and producing energy.

HOW DO WE FIX THIS?

The first step toward optimal digestive health is to have a look at the food you eat. You need to include foods in your diet that are as close to natural as possible. If something has a whole list of ingredients that you cannot pronounce, it should not make it into your shopping cart.

Better to stick to natural, whole foods from organic sources. Grass-fed, naturally raised beef is an example of the type of meat you should be looking for. If you have the space, try your hand at growing your own organic fruit or veggies.

Adding extra fiber to your diet and reducing the amount of sugar and chemicals you take in will go a long way to restoring your digestive health. With ACV, you can give the microflora in your system a boost and help to improve the absorption of nutrients from your food. ACV has several beneficial effects when it comes to the digestive tract and helping improve nutrient absorption.

ACV SLOWS DOWN HOW FAST THE STOMACH EMPTIES

Your food takes some time to digest in the stomach. The stomach acid and digestive enzymes need time to break down the food you eat. The problem is that the different types of foods are emptied at different rates.

Proteins are moved along at the fastest rates, with carbs coming a close second. Fats are held in the stomach for longer, and so are foods that are high in fiber. Our typical Western diets includes a lot of fat but also a lot of protein and carbs. Most of us are not eating nearly enough fiber. Fibrous foods include fresh vegetables and fruits, as well as legumes and some grains like quinoa, which contains twice as much fiber as most other grains.

Basically, the food we are eating tends to be passed along to the digestive system before it should be. It is like the stomach is saying, "I give up, you clean up this mess!"

Studies have shown that ACV helps to inhibit amylases, the enzymes that break down carbs and delay the rate at which the stomach empties. The natural acidity of ACV plays a further role in this process. Put very simply, receptors present in the duodenum of the small intestine will gauge the acidity of the food.

If that food is deemed too acidic, these receptors will signal the stomach so that the process of gastric emptying is delayed. The more acidic the food, the longer it will stay in the stomach and the more time the stomach enzymes and acids have to break it down.

That said, the acetic acid in ACV is mild enough that it won't delay the process too much. If the process is slowed down too much, this could also be problematic and manifest in symptoms like bloating, belching, and acid reflux.

REDUCES THE BUILDUP OF GLUCOSE IN THE BLOOD AFTER THE MEAL

The type of food you eat will determine whether your blood sugar spikes after eating. The easier the food is to digest, the more glucose hits your blood and the more likely it is that the levels will spike dangerously.

Studies have shown that ingesting a few teaspoons of ACV with your meals can result in a reduction in the buildup of glucose after the meal of around 20 percent. This is quite a significant change and is of special interest to those with diabetes or prediabetes.

It is also helpful if you have been eating simpler carbs. That said, it is not a magic bullet. You still need to be conscious of what you are eating. Nothing can stop the sugar spike if you are eating six candy bars, for example.

IMPROVES INSULIN SENSITIVITY

Further studies have shown that ACV can improve insulin sensitivity by as much as 34 percent when you are eating a high-carb meal. What that means is that ACV actually helps to make the insulin in your body work more efficiently.

HELPS YOU FEEL FULLER

Many studies indicate that vinegar is useful in helping you to feel fuller. On average, it was found that those who ate vinegar with a high-carb meal tended to eat up to about 275 fewer calories throughout the rest of the day.

We all know that taking in fewer calories helps us to lose weight if we tend to overeat. Even more important, it was found that those individuals who took 1 tablespoon of vinegar a day lost, on average, 2.6 pounds over a 12-week period and showed a reduction in belly fat and triglycerides as well. Those taking double that amount lost, on average, 3.7 pounds over the same 12-week period. Now, that may not sound like an awful lot, but considering that the only change they made to their lifestyle was consuming vinegar every day, it is quite an interesting statistic.

CAN HELP IN REDUCING INFLAMMATION

ACV is very useful for the good microbes in the gut, as they can feed on the pectin in it. ACV itself contains beneficial bacteria that can help bolster the good bacteria in your gut. The acetic acid in the vinegar helps to suppress protein that may promote inflammation, and it helps kill off harmful bacteria.

It is also useful in killing off food-borne bacteria. If you are at a restaurant and are not sure how sanitary it is, drinking ACV with your meal will help to destroy food-borne pathogens. You can also take advantage of this quality when preparing food at home. You can soak or wash your fruits and vegetables in a mixture of one part of ACV to four parts of water to help kill off any pathogens that might be present.

IMPROVES THE ABSORPTION
OF MINERALS FROM FOOD

Dr. Hans Adolf Krebs earned a Nobel Prize for his theory on the citric acid cycle. Krebs found that the nutrients in our food must be combined with acetic acid in order to be properly broken down and used. ACV contains the acetic acid necessary to complete the citric acid cycle. Therefore, taking ACV with meals will help our bodies to better absorb the nutrients and minerals in our food.

As we get older, our bodies are not as effective at absorbing minerals such as iron and calcium from the food we eat. ACV helps with this by mixing the minerals with other compounds so that the end result is more easily absorbed.

Are you ready to start getting your daily dose of ACV? There are a few ways to do this. A simple one is to mix 1 tablespoon of ACV in a glass of water and drink it down 15 minutes before each meal.

However, that is not very appetizing. What you can do instead is start incorporating it into your meal plan. Below we have three easy recipes to get you started.

ACV BEET SALAD

Serves 2

You can whip up this salad in minutes, and it tastes great, to boot. The beets are loaded with iron that is much more easily absorbed because of the ACV. This salad is packed with nutrients and fiber that will give you tons of energy. The ginger, ACV, and olive oil have potent anti-inflammatory effects as well.

1 teaspoon honey

1 tablespoon ACV

½ teaspoon fresh ginger, peeled and grated

1 teaspoon extra virgin olive oil

½ cup grated beet roots

½ cup Granny Smith apple, grated, with the peel on

½ cup carrots, peeled and grated

2 teaspoons parsley, chopped

Mix together the honey, ACV, ginger, and olive oil, and set aside. Mix together the beat roots, apple, carrots, and parsley. Stir in the dressing. Refrigerate for about 30 minutes to let the flavors develop.

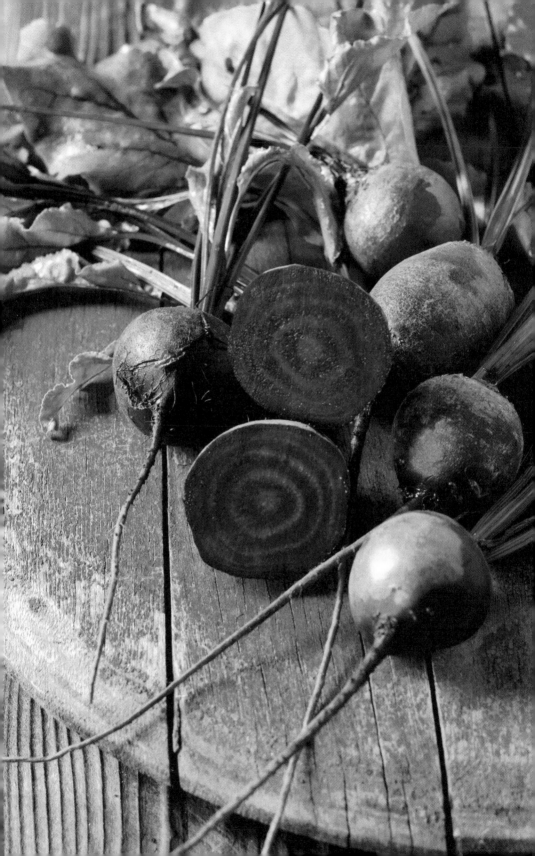

ACV SUPERFOOD SALAD

Serves 2

Use the power of ACV to help you absorb all the plentiful nutrients contained in this health-boosting salad!

3 cups romaine lettuce

1 cup arugula

1 cup raw kale, chopped

½ cup watercress

½ cup red cabbage, chopped

¼ cup sprouted mung or adzuki beans

¼ cup shelled edamame

¼ cup shredded green cabbage

¼ cup broccoli sprouts

3 tablespoons raw pumpkin seeds

1 tablespoon raw chia seeds

¼ cup pomegranate seeds

2 tablespoons sorrel leaf, chopped

3 tablespoons nasturtium flower petals

1 tablespoon walnuts, chopped

1 tablespoon nasturtium leaves, chopped

4 tablespoons cold-pressed olive oil

3 tablespoons ACV

½ teaspoon Celtic sea salt

½ teaspoon powdered turmeric

¼ teaspoon powdered cumin

Toss all ingredients together and serve immediately.

WARMING ACV HONEY SPREAD

Serves 2

- ½ cup chilled ghee (clarified butter)
- ¼ cup chilled raw honey
- ½ teaspoon ACV
- ⅛ teaspoon powdered ginger
- ⅛ teaspoon cardamom
- ⅛ teaspoon nutmeg
- ⅛ teaspoon cinnamon

Blend all ingredients gently with a wooden spoon until thoroughly mixed. Serve as a spread on sprouted grain toast, muffins, rice cakes, or crackers. Can also be mixed with granola or cereal. Or use to top yogurt. Store in the refrigerator.

KALE-STRAWBERRY SMOOTHIE

Serves 2

This is perfect for mornings when you need something to get you going. The kale is rich in iron, and its absorption is facilitated by the ACV. The banana gives the smoothie a lovely sweet flavor and is a great source of potassium.

1 ripe banana, peeled and frozen

1 cup frozen strawberries

¾ cups curly kale, without the stems

¾ cup spinach

½ cup carrots, chopped

1 tablespoon fresh mint

1 teaspoon ACV

1 scoop of your favorite protein powder (optional)

Put all ingredients into a blender with 1 cup of water. Blend until it is a drinkable consistency, adding more water if needed.

WATERMELON ACV SPRITZ

Serves 8

This makes a big pitcher that is perfect for when you have friends over.
It tastes so good they won't even know how healthy it is. It is also a great way
for you to get some ACV into your diet.

 8 cups carbonated spring water

 1 cup seeded and cubed watermelon

 1 cucumber, sliced

 Juice and pulp of 1 lime

 2 tablespoons ACV

Mix all the ingredients together and refrigerate. Take out the watermelon
cubes just before you serve it.

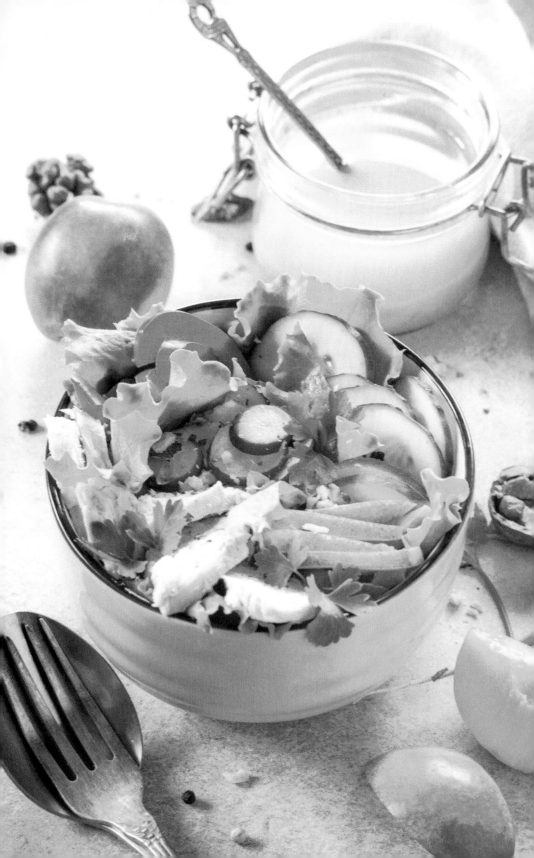

Chapter 8

Healthy Cholesterol and Insulin Levels Using Apple Cider Vinegar

Organic ACV left in its unfiltered, unadulterated, and unrefined state retains its optimum health-promoting properties. It has been used for thousands of years to treat all sorts of ailments and diseases. In unfiltered organic ACV, a beneficial group of bacteria and acids remains and creates the murky web-like mother. The mother also allows the vinegar to get stronger over time and maintain its beneficial probiotic and immune-boosting properties. To get the most out of using ACV, make sure you buy it raw and with the mother intact.

The best is a cloudy vinegar that still contains the beneficial compounds and friendly enzymes and bacteria that promote healing. It is loaded with pectin and minerals like potassium, magnesium, sodium, and calcium. It also contains vitamins and beta-carotene. Beta-carotene is supposed to help people retain their youth longer, as it counters the damage caused by free radicals. Experiments have proven that ACV also contains carbolic acids, aldehydes, ketones, and acetates. The potassium present is crucial as it helps in the removal of excess water and toxic waste in the system. Calcium, which is important for the bones and for osteoporosis resistance, is another important constituent of ACV.

SUPPORTS HEART HEALTH

Studies have shown that the consumption of ACV helps support heart health and that it is very effective in reducing the risk of heart disease.

Acetic acid created in the fermentation of ACV has a wide array of health benefits. Certain pharmaceutical medications contain acetic acid in concentrated form. Studies have looked at the role of acetic acid in lowering and regulating blood pressure and have found it to be beneficial.

In a 12-week study from 2009, the researchers found that consuming ACV significantly lowered triglycerides and blood pressure. As we all know, heart disease is still one of the leading causes of death in the world. Several measurable biological factors either decrease or increase the probability of cardiovascular disease. Studies conducted on rats have found that several of these risk factors improve with the consumption of ACV. Studies on humans still have to be conducted to understand the beneficial effects of consuming ACV on heart health; however, encouraging studies on animals indicate that ACV is useful for a variety of health concerns.

ACV also contains magnesium, which relaxes blood vessels. It also lowers high blood pressure and helps keep it within healthy limits. Its high potassium values help to balance out sodium levels in the body, which aid in maintaining optimal blood pressure. When you are taking ACV, it is beneficial to also cut down on your overall sodium intake.

IMPROVES CHOLESTEROL

Recent studies have shown that ACV helps improve cholesterol levels. Acetic acid in its concentrated form has been studied to observe its role in the dissolving of cholesterol deposits in the arteries.

ACV contains chlorogenic acid, which is an antioxidant. It has been shown to prevent LDL cholesterol particles from being oxidized, a crucial step in preventing the development of heart disease. LDL cholesterol creates fatty buildup in arteries that can narrow them, potentially leading to a variety of health problems. The pectin in the apples attaches itself to cholesterol globules. Some studies performed on rats have shown ACV's ability to lower blood pressure. Human studies still need to take place, but the prospects are hopeful.

The water-soluble fiber pectin is present in ACV. Pectin eliminates and absorbs fats and cholesterol from the body. Additionally, the amino acids in ACV work to counterbalance oxidized LDL cholesterol. ACV is a robust antioxidant.

Researchers from Mizkan, a Japanese food manufacturer, conducted a study the found that regular daily vinegar intake significantly lowers the level of LDL cholesterol in blood samples.

BALANCES BLOOD SUGAR

Medical research has found that the acetic acid found in ACV can balance and lower blood sugar, plus improve insulin sensitivity and insulin responses. It lowers blood sugar levels and helps keep blood sugar in check. ACV has myriad benefits for insulin function and regulating blood sugar levels.

A research team from Arizona State University recently found that drinking ACV regularly moderates the rise of blood sugar after high-carbohydrate meals. They found that it reduces blood sugar by 34 percent when eating 50 grams of white bread.

INSULIN SENSITIVITY

ACV has numerous benefits for insulin function. It improves insulin sensitivity during a high-carb meal by 19–34 percent and significantly lowers blood glucose and insulin responses.

TYPE 2 DIABETES

In the next 25 years the number of Americans with type 2 diabetes is expected to increase by 50 percent. Type 2 diabetes is characterized by elevated blood glucose levels, either because of insulin resistance or the inability to produce insulin.

A recent study showed that ACV weakened the glucose and insulin responses to a sucrose or starch load—this means that it's possible that it can delay or prevent the onset of type 2 diabetes in high-risk populations. In yet another report, researchers found vinegar to be effective in reducing postprandial glycemia and insulinemia in people with varying degrees of insulin sensitivity. In other words, ACV can alleviate the harmful effects of diabetes.

It has been found that ACV consumption increases insulin-stimulated glucose uptake tested via the forearm muscle in people with type 2 diabetes.

Elevated blood sugar levels can be an issue even when diabetes is not present and can lead to aging and increase risks for chronic diseases. It was found in various studies that ingesting ACV reduced blood glucose concentrations in healthy adults and in otherwise healthy adults diagnosed with prediabetes.

One of the older and most effective ways of controlling your blood sugar is through diet, limiting your intake (or avoiding altogether) refined carbohydrates and sugar. Incorporating ACV into your diet along with these steps is a great way to regulate your blood sugar.

To slow down the rise of blood sugar, 2 minutes before a meal drink 1 tablespoon of ACV in a glass of water, or add 1 tablespoon of ACV to your salads. This helps regulate your blood sugar levels after your meal.

To improve insulin function and balance blood sugar levels, before bedtime drink 1 tablespoon of ACV in a glass of water. It has been found that drinking ACV before bed can reduce fasting blood sugars by 4 percent.

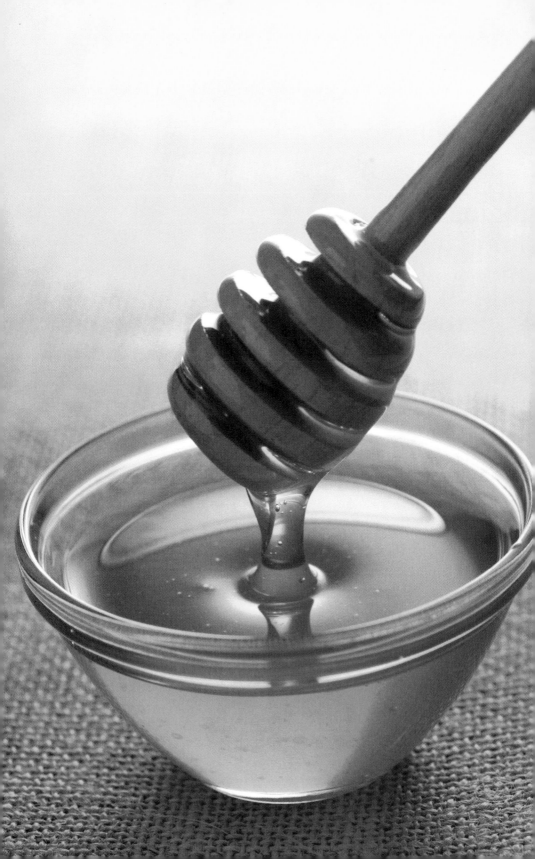

ACV AND HONEY MIX

Serves 1

This recipe is designed to lower your sodium levels. ACV and honey both have potassium, which balance out the sodium in your body and lower your blood pressure. They both also contain magnesium, which relaxes your blood vessels and also lowers blood pressure.

    1 tablespoon ACV

    1 tablespoon raw organic honey

Mix the ACV and honey into 4 ounces of water. Drink twice a day in place of other recommended daily ACV drinks. Choose up to two ways per day to consume your ACV drinks.

ACV SALAD DRESSING

This is a great recipe for high blood pressure. Fresh veggies increase the amount of fiber, vitamins, minerals, and antioxidants in your diet. And all these contribute to lower blood pressure. The ACV gives you a shot of extra potassium, which keeps sodium levels balanced.

¼ cup ACV

¼ cup extra virgin olive oil

Juice of 1 lemon

½ teaspoon dried basil or dill weed

1 teaspoon mustard powder

Salt and pepper, to taste

Combine all ingredients in a lidded jar. Close the jar and shake well. Drizzle 2 tablespoons over a salad.

ACV CAYENNE PEPPER TONIC

Serves 1

Cayenne pepper and ACV both work to lower blood pressure.

    1 tablespoon ACV

    Pinch cayenne pepper

Mix the ACV and pepper into a glass of water. Take this twice a day in place of other recommended daily ACV doses. As you get comfortable with the spiciness of it, increase the amount of cayenne little by little until you reach $^1/_4$ teaspoon.

To lower your cholesterol, mix 1 tablespoon ACV in a glass of water 15 minutes before each meal every day. Pectin is a water-soluble fiber found in ACV. It eliminates cholesterol from the body. You can maximize this benefit by adding extra fiber-rich food to your diet and drinking extra water each day.

HONEY-COCONUT CHOLESTEROL BUSTER

Serves 1

  1 tablespoon pure organic coconut oil

  1 tablespoon raw organic honey

  2 teaspoons ACV

  5 teaspoons aloe vera gel

Mix the coconut oil and honey into a small quantity of hot water, until well combined. Stir this mixture into 8 ounces of water, along with the ACV and aloe. Try to drink it fairly quickly; do not sip it. Drink once a day.

POWERHOUSE CHOLESTEROL BUSTER

Serves 5

> 1 cup lemon juice
>
> 1 cup ginger juice
>
> 1 cup ACV
>
> 3 cups organic raw honey

Combine the lemon juice and ginger juice in a saucepan, and bring to a boil. Reduce the heat to a simmer, and cook until reduced to 1 cup. Add the ACV and honey, and stir well to combine. Drink 3 tablespoons of this mixture in 4 ounces of water on an empty stomach daily.

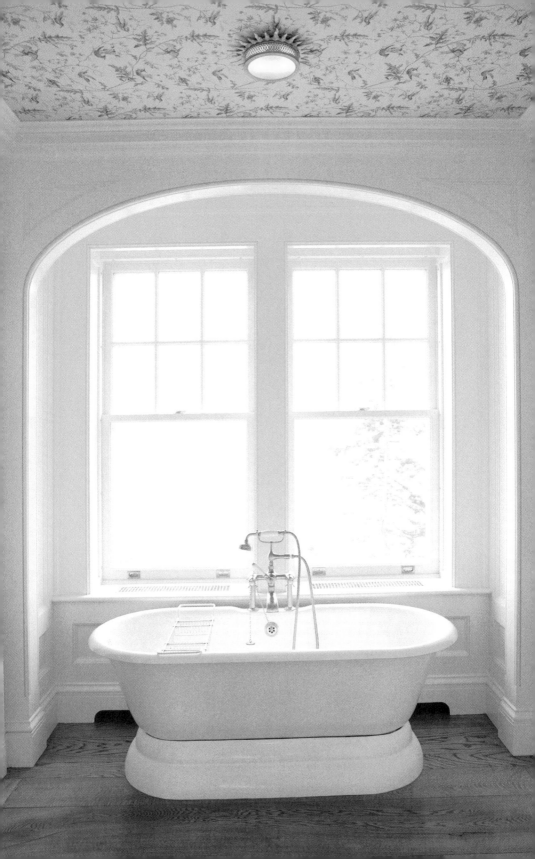

Chapter 9

Apple Cider Vinegar's Prebiotics and Treatments for Candida

ACV is so much more than a delicious addition to a recipe. There are multiple health benefits from consuming and applying diluted ACV. Put away that salad dressing bottle and take a look at what else this vinegar has to offer.

ACV contains the ingredient pectin. Pectin is both a helpful prebiotic, which supports the growth of healthy bacteria, and a probiotic—the living bacteria that greatly benefit your overall health. Prebiotics and probiotics play a role in aiding gastrointestinal wellness and can even benefit the immune system by promoting pathogen destruction in the digestive tract. Consuming ACV can help support both your digestive and immune systems by acting as a prebiotic and supporting healthy probiotic growth. Prebiotics are food for probiotics.

ACV is acidic, which can help in instances where your body's pH is too alkaline. The pH scale, which indicates alkalinity and acidity, ranges from 0 to 14, with 0 being the most acidic and 14 being the most alkaline, or basic. A healthy pH can help maintain the balance of good and bad bacteria in your body.

Yeast infections and bacterial vaginosis are problems that occur when your vagina's pH becomes too alkaline. The vagina is naturally acidic due to the presence of healthy bacteria living in the vagina that produce acids that keep the levels of unhealthy bacteria down. A normal pH level for your vagina should be between 3.8 and 4.5. If the pH level starts to increase above 4.5, the healthy bacterial flora in your vaginal tract will decline and the bad bacteria such as *Gardnerella vaginalis* will increase.

A variety of factors might cause your vagina to start turning too alkaline. Menstrual blood can push your vagina toward basic because blood has a neutral pH of 7. Male ejaculate can also throw things out of order because semen is more alkaline on the pH scale. So are many of the soaps or vaginal "cleansers" you might find at a store. Antibiotics can wipe out all the healthy bacteria along with the bad. Diet can also come into play, as too much sugar and gluten can knock pH out of balance.

If you're familiar with your vagina, you'll notice the moment it begins to turn alkaline. Your vagina will feel off and smell different, and the consistency of the discharge will change. However, if you're unsure, you can test your vaginal pH at home with a pH test strip from your local drugstore. You can also be on the lookout for the following symptoms to know when something just isn't right. Symptoms of a yeast infection include itchy labia (vaginal lips), itching inside your vagina, a thick white discharge like cottage cheese, a burning sensation inside your vagina, and pain during sex or urination. Bacterial vaginosis symptoms are similar. They include vaginal itching and a thin gray or white discharge accompanied with a fishy odor, but no pain with sex or urination.

ACV can help bring your pH back to a more acidic level. Its acidic qualities help to destroy any bad bacteria causing trouble in your vagina and tip the pH scale back to acid. The prebiotic pectin in the vinegar will also help restore the growth of healthy bacteria.

There are some important things to note before you try any of the recipes in this chapter. For starters, it's important to use organic ACV. Non-organic ACV has been pasteurized to produce a clearer, more attractive-looking fluid, but this removes all the beneficial probiotic bacteria that we're looking for. Look for organic ACV with the mother, the source of the cloudiness in the vinegar, intact. It might not look attractive, but it contains the beneficial qualities that will help bring you some relief.

PATCH TEST

It is important to dilute the vinegar you use. Using straight ACV could produce an irritating sensation and can be too much. Dilute the vinegar with water and other ingredients as directed in these recipes and patch test in the case of external applications to see if you need to dilute the vinegar a little more. In the case of an ingested remedy, rinse your mouth out with water afterward to avoid any enamel wear on your teeth.

A patch test is applying a little bit of a topical recipe to the inside of your arm and waiting 2 minutes to make sure there is no irritation. Then you can go ahead and use the rest knowing that the ingredients agree with your individual bodily systems.

ACV BATH

Yields 1 bath

An ACV bath can help treat infection, provide relief to any irritation at the infection site, and deodorize.

 2 cups organic ACV

Fill the bathtub. Add the ACV and stir to dilute. Do a patch test for sensitivity, and add more water if irritation occurs. When the mixture is just right, climb in and sit with your knees drawn up to your chest for 15–20 minutes. When you're done soaking, carefully pat yourself dry before putting on a pair of cotton underwear. You can use a hair dryer on a cool setting to gently dry yourself off. Try this bath once a day until symptoms subside.

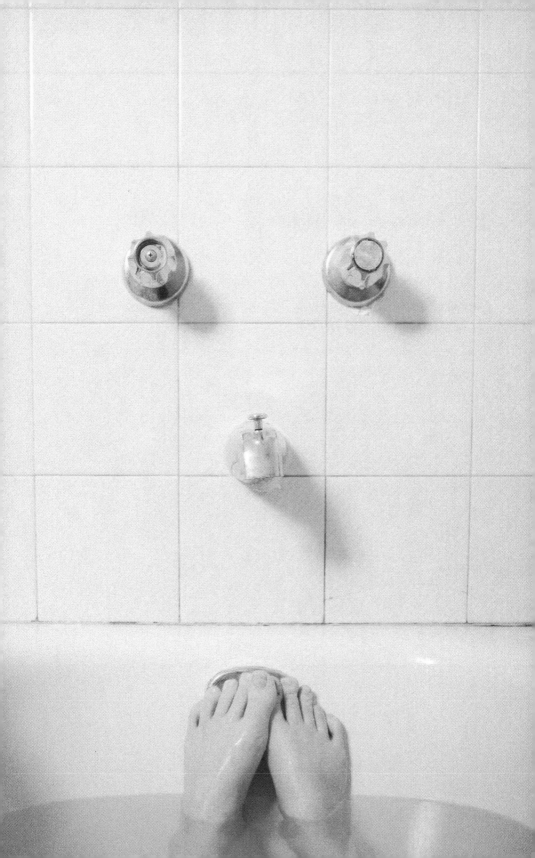

APPLE CIDER VINEGAR SPRAY

Yields about ⅔ cup

An ACV spray can be helpful for mild, external symptoms of infection.

    10 tablespoons distilled water
    1 tablespoon organic ACV

Combine the water and ACV in a spray bottle. Shake the spray bottle to combine, do a patch test for sensitivity, and add more water if irritation occurs. When the mixture is to your liking, spray on the infected area and wait for it to completely dry before putting on a pair of cotton underwear. Use this spray as needed. Store it in the refrigerator for an added cooling sensation.

ACV TOWEL SOAK

Yields about ⅔ cup

> 10 tablespoons distilled water
>
> 1 tablespoon organic ACV

In a bowl, combine the water and ACV. Do a patch test for sensitivity, and add more water if irritation occurs. When the mixture is to your liking, soak a hand towel in the mixture, and wring out the excess liquid. Place it on the infection site and let it sit for 15 minutes. When the 15 minutes are up, remove the towel and let the area dry completely before putting on a pair of cotton underwear.

ACV TONIC

Serves 1

ACV will also help restore your pH balance when taken internally and can be used as a preventive. It supports healthy digestion and a strong immune system, and can even help you fall asleep when taken before bed.

> 1 tablespoon organic ACV
>
> Honey

Combine the ACV with the honey in 8 ounces of warm water. Drink twice a day. Be sure to rinse your mouth with water afterward to keep the acidic vinegar from wearing down your tooth enamel.

Those without vaginas can also be affected by infections from unbalanced pH. Sexual intercourse with someone with a yeast infection, for example, can spread the infection to the penis. Symptoms can include itching, burning, redness at the tip, and painful urination. These symptoms can be similar to those of STDs, so it is important to get tested before moving forward with any of the treatments previously described. If you're certain you don't have an STD, try the above treatments. You can also use this recipe for more direct treatment of the penis.

APPLE CIDER VINEGAR COTTON BALL TREATMENT

Yields 2 quarts

> 2 quarts warm distilled water
>
> 2 tablespoons organic ACV

Combine the water and ACV. Perform a patch test for sensitivity, and add more water if irritation occurs. Dip a cotton ball or pad into the liquid and gently bathe the affected area. Use this method twice a day to treat the infection.

You should expect to see results from these treatments within a few days or weeks, as everybody has a different capacity for healing. The symptoms may worsen at first, but should subside after a few days. You can support these treatments by consuming probiotic-rich foods like yogurt and avoiding excess sugar in your diet. You can also take probiotics in the form of supplements. Wear cotton underwear and try to keep your genitals cool and dry. Sleeping without underwear can help.

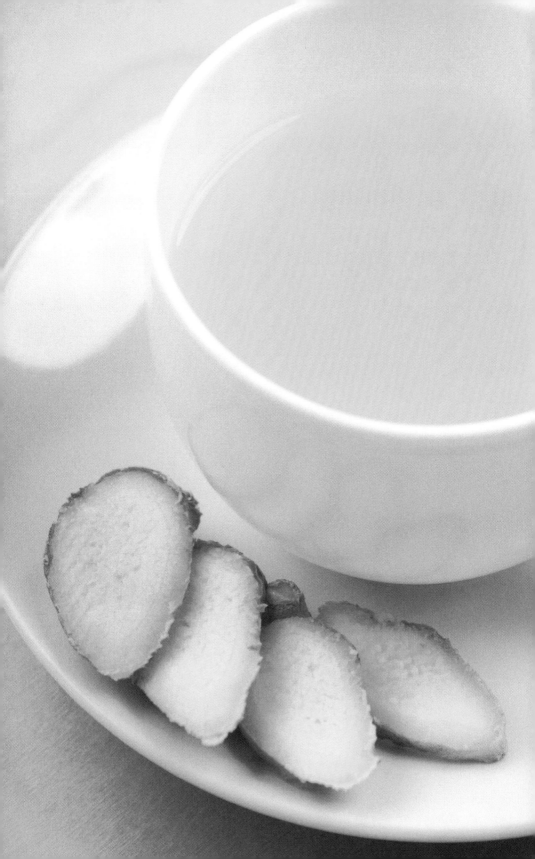

Chapter 10

Curing Heartburn and Other Digestive Uses

That painful flaming sensation in your chest known as gastroesophageal reflux disease (more commonly known as heartburn, or acid reflux) usually occurs when your bodily functions are out of balance. That burning sensation generally sits in the upper chest or upper abdomen. It may feel like heat, but actually it's gastric, or stomach, acid.

How the body breaks down food and converts it to energy is a pretty complicated process. The digestive enzymes in our gut move toward the food we eat. They then encapsulate and break it down so our body can use it for energy. When we do something extreme, like binging on sausage pizza in front of the television at midnight before falling asleep, the gastric acid moves from our stomach to underneath the breastbone and causes us discomfort.

Gastric acid is really tough stuff. Something has to break down all that food, right? Gastric acid is made for the digestive system, which has a protective lining that helps keep this powerful substance only where it is meant to be. When gastric acid travels up the esophagus instead of staying down in the gut breaking food into amino acids, that's where that painful sensation comes in.

We know that heartburn is caused by elevated gastric acid. But what elevates it? What makes it rise in our esophagus and give us that painful burning that forces us to seek relief as soon as possible?

Eating plays a part in causing heartburn. Eating processed and acidic foods can overwhelm the stomach. Food sensitivities also play a part. Green peppers are a common cause of heartburn. Late-night eating can also play a part.

Healthy eating habits are the first treatment for heartburn. Most doctors recommend a diet rich in fruit and vegetables and low in processed foods. Our bodies need fresh fruits and vegetables that are rich in nutrients and the fiber our body requires to function. Eliminating food that is highly processed for the majority of meals will help calm heartburn.

Remember how at summer camp we were made to relax after a meal? Well, it turns out that wasn't just the counselor trying to get a break or a nap in before the next activity. The best way to prevent heartburn after a meal is to do not too little and not too much. Lying down can cause it. Overexertion can cause it. Your best bet is the practice moderate exertion after a meal. That can be a light walk or an hour or so in front of the television or with your nose in a book.

It's not just the timing of food, but the type. If you are trying to prevent heartburn, it is best to avoid high-fat and fried food. Tomatoes and tomato products should be avoided in addition to citrus foods like oranges and pineapple. Water should be the only beverage you drink, as alcohol and coffee can aggravate a heartburn condition. You should be eating lots of fruits and vegetables in variety. That might mean a day of cucumbers, strawberries, and carrots, followed the next day with an avocado salad. Top that salad with a vinaigrette made with apple cider vinegar, and you've got a recipe for heartburn prevention.

Heartburn can also be caused by being overweight and/or stressed. It's important to manage your weight and to practice exercises like yoga or stretching that help you cope with the stress of life. Being anxious can also cause heartburn. Finding ways to alleviate the symptoms of anxiety can also help prevent this condition. If you can, get out in nature, take a nice long walk, and experience a walking meditation. Think mindful, positive thoughts while you cook some yummy veggies like zucchini on the grill with a side of peaches. Consume those foods with an ACV tonic. It will be delicious and nutritious and aid your body in healing your weakened gut muscles.

ACIDIC VERSUS ALKALINE

Foods like tomatoes, green peppers, red meats, poultry, and fish are acidic. Dairy, eggs, and grains are also considered acidic. They are represented by the vinegar in a science fair volcano.

Alkaline foods or foods that represent the baking soda in our model volcano are fruits, nuts, legumes, and vegetables. A healthy person can eat both, and both have nutritional value. However, someone who is recovering from a heartburn condition might likely want to avoid too many foods on the acidic list. She will want to be practicing mindful healthy eating habits.

Mindful eating is eating with intention and being present to the sensations your body is experiencing while you eat the food. What it feels like to chew, the taste, the aroma, and the way the food looks are all things you can notice when you eat mindfully. When you do anything mindfully, that gives you the opportunity to slow down. So eating mindfully means you'll eat more slowly. You'll experience less stress. You won't be watching TV or looking at your phone or doing things that speed up your mind, which causes anxiety. That anxiety can cause heartburn and poor digestion. It is better for your health to slow down and chew your food thoroughly. A side benefit is that when you eat more slowly and mindfully, you will consume only what your body is hungry for because you will notice that you're full instead of overeating. Overeating is also a cause of heartburn.

We live in a fast-paced world and we need to slow down in many areas of our lives. Many people end up eating over the sink as they rush from one task to another or out the door for work or to drive their children to baseball practice. It is uncommon now for people to sit down and have a relaxed social meal where they are not doing something else at the same time. But that is not how our bodies were wired to consume food. We are wired to mindfully consume food, whether alone or in a social setting where we might talk and interact, but the only other thing we're doing is eating.

So, isn't this book about ACV? How are we supposed to eat it and still avoid acid?

The comparison between acids and food is just to draw out the distinction. Did you know that some types of heartburn can actually be prevented by imbibing vinegar?

ACV isn't a typical vinegar. It is acidic like other vinegars, but it is an all-natural vinegar that is made from the fermentation of apples. As the apples ferment, they leave behind what is called the mother of the apple.

This mother is a smooth substance that is found at the bottom of the container or jar used to ferment the apples. It is filmy and has the consistency of a cobweb. Many people love this mother and eat it almost daily as a way to practice good eating health.

The mother contains enzymes, protein, and pectin. People who brew this type of vinegar frequently eat the mother.

ACV doesn't have any major side effects; it can't hurt you if used within the established safety parameters. Like anything else, of course, you should consume it in moderation. Most people who use it down at least 1 tablespoon of ACV per day.

The natural acids in the ACV go into your stomach and balance the acids already present there. Adding ACV to your diet causes an increase of acid, forcing your own body to develop neutralizers that remedy it. When you accidentally overeat or eat late at night and then fall asleep, your body will be better equipped to deal with it.

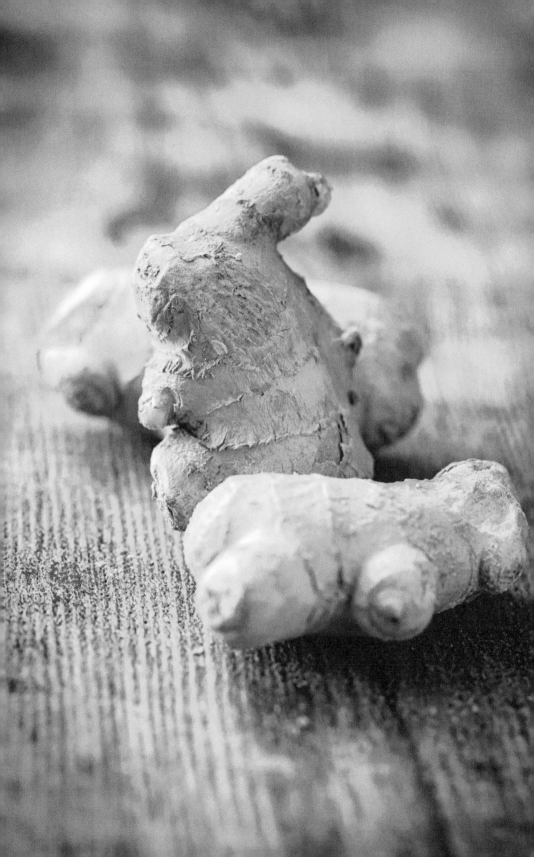

ACV GINGER TUMMY SOOTHER

Serves 1

    4 cups water

    ¼ teaspoon ACV

    3-inch piece ginger, coarsely chopped (not peeled)

    1 tablespoon lemon zest

    1 tablespoon fennel seed

Place all ingredients in a saucepan and simmer for 30 minutes. Strain out solid ingredients and consume liquid—can be served warm or at room temperature.

ANTI-HEARTBURN GINGER TEA

Serves 1

Take this in the morning. to prevent heartburn later. This will boost your brain and pump you up.

    ¼ teaspoon ginger

    1 tablespoon ACV

    1 green tea bag

Mix together the ginger and vinegar, and let the tea bag rest in it for a few minutes. Take as a shot or add to water.

ACV ENERGY BOOSTING CLEANSING SLAW

Serves 2

> 2 cups green cabbage, chopped
>
> 2 cups red cabbage, chopped
>
> 2 cups carrot, shredded
>
> ½ cup parsley, chopped
>
> 1 teaspoon lemon juice
>
> 1 teaspoon ACV
>
> 1 teaspoon flaxseed oil
>
> ½ teaspoon fennel seed
>
> ⅛ teaspoon Celtic sea salt
>
> ⅛ teaspoon cumin
>
> Dash black pepper (optional)

Stir all ingredients and serve cold to revitalize your digestive and endocrine systems. This cleansing veggie blast contains lots of fiber to clear out any proverbial digestive cobwebs. It also has hormone-regulating properties due to its high proportion of cruciferous cabbage containing DIM (diindolylmethane). And it packs a powerful nutritional punch.

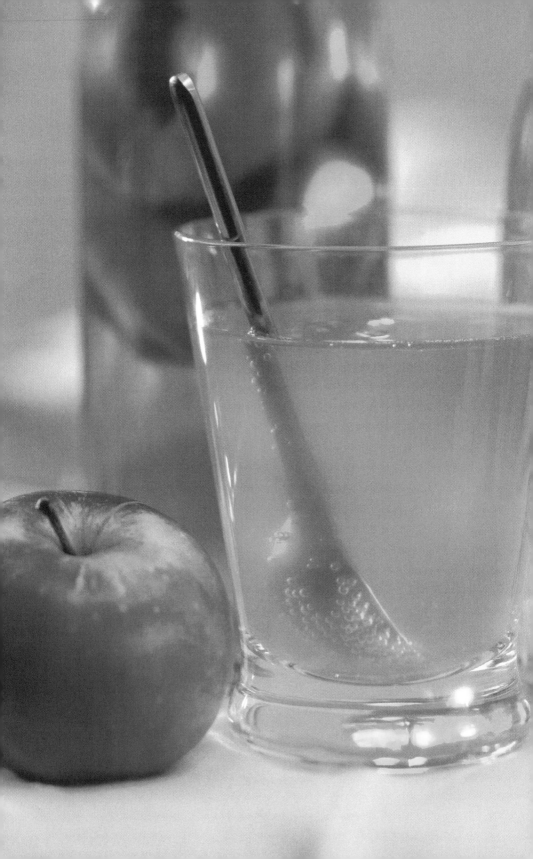

HEARTBURN CLEANSING DRINK

Serves 1

This fresh tasting detox drink has diuretic and cleansing benefits. Drink this drink at any time during the day.

2 tablespoons ACV

1 tablespoon lemon juice

⅛ cup fresh parsley, chopped

1 teaspoon raw local honey

Combine all ingredients in 12–16 ounces of hot water, cover, and steep for 5 to 10 minutes.

BEST HERBS FOR HEARTBURN

These herbs can be taken in tea form. Add a splash of ACV to gently calm your digestive system.

Lemon balm

Marshmallow Root

German Chamomile

Licorice

Spearmint

Peppermint

Slippery Elm Bark

Ginger

Basil

Also consider adding digestive-enzyme supplements to your diet. Oftentimes, we are underproducing these crucial compounds and we simply need a boost to support our digestion.

HEARTBURN PREVENTION APPLE CIDER VINEGAR DRESSING

Serves 1

This is the tastiest and easiest way to get your daily dose of ACV. If eaten with a meal it will prevent heartburn.

>   2 tablespoons olive oil
>
>   1½ tablespoons ACV
>
>   1 teaspoon mustard powder
>
>   1 teaspoon ginger powder
>
>   1 teaspoon dried chives

Combine all ingredients in a jar, and set aside. After a couple hours, pour over your favorite salad.

GINGER-LIME ICE POPS

Serves 4

1 medium-sized lime

2 tablespoons ginger juice (premade or freshly juiced)

Whole leaves from ¼ bunch fresh mint

¼ teaspoon ACV

¼ teaspoon powdered stevia

Make lime puree for pops by peeling one medium-sized lime and blending it in a food processor on low for 30 seconds. Stir all ingredients together and pour into ice pop molds. Freeze and enjoy.

FENNEL BULB SPREAD

Serves 4

> 3 tablespoons coconut oil
>
> 1 large fennel bulb (remove stalks)
>
> ¼ teaspoon ACV
>
> ½ teaspoon coriander
>
> ¼ teaspoon cumin
>
> ½ cup artichoke hearts, in brine
>
> 1 teaspoon fennel seeds
>
> Toast points (for serving)
>
> ¼ bunch chopped fresh dill (as garnish)

Place the coconut oil in a warm skillet. Sauté all ingredients, except the toast points and the dill, until soft. Remove from heat and let cool. Pour contents of pan into a food processor and blend until smooth. Serve in a decorative dish with toast points and garnish with fresh dill.

NO-SUGAR HONEY-MUSTARD HORSERADISH SAUCE

Serves 4

    4 cups sheep or Greek-style yogurt

    1 tablespoon horseradish powder

    1 tablespoon mustard powder

    ¼ teaspoon ACV

    Juice of half a lemon

    2 teaspoons sea salt

    1 bunch fresh chives, chopped

    ¼ teaspoon powdered stevia

    Several dashes freshly ground black pepper to taste

Whisk all ingredients together until smooth. Serve chilled over fish or chicken or as a dip with fresh vegetables.

PECORINO PEAR SALAD

Serves 4

- 4 cups arugula
- 2 cups chopped watercress
- ½ cup pistachio kernels, lightly salted
- ½ cup pecorino cheese, grated
- ½ cup pear, finely chopped (with skin)
- 4 tablespoons pistachio oil
- 1½ tablespoons ACV
- ¼ cup, fresh mint leaves, chopped
- Dash fresh ground black pepper

Toss all ingredients together and serve immediately.

FENNEL CASHEW "CHEEZE" PESTO

Serves 4

   3 cups raw cashews

   ¼ cup fennel seeds

   1 tablespoon mustard powder

   ½ teaspoon sea salt

   1 tablespoon dried chives

   ¼ teaspoon ACV

Blend all ingredients in food processor until pulverized except for the ACV. Remove from food processor and place in a dish, add ACV and water as needed for desired consistency.

TANGY CHAI ALMONDS

Serves 4

6 cups raw almonds

½ teaspoon powdered ginger

½ teaspoon powdered cloves

½ teaspoon coriander

½ teaspoon cardamom

½ teaspoon nutmeg

½ teaspoon cinnamon

1 tablespoon coconut oil

1 tablespoon ACV

Toss almonds and other ingredients in a mixing bowl. Spread in a single layer on a baking sheet. Bake at 350°F for 20 minutes, gently stirring after 10 minutes. Serve warm.

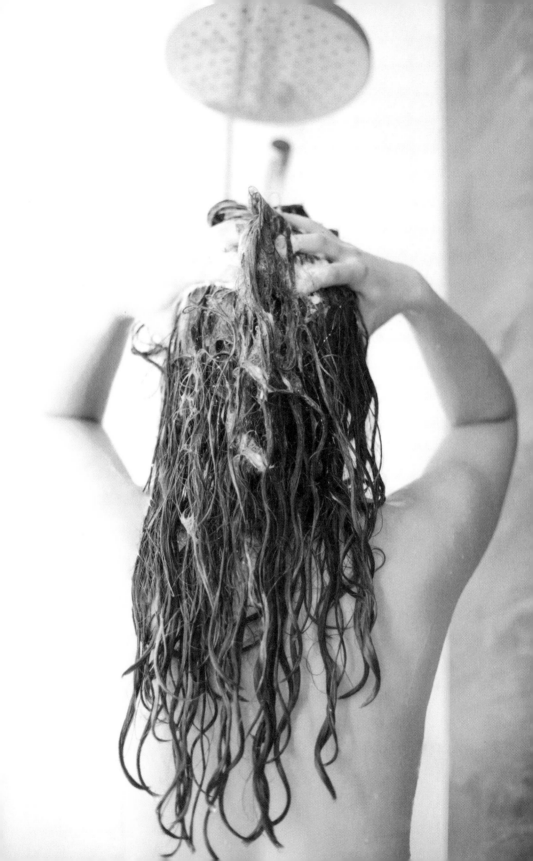

Chapter 11

Lustrous Skin and Hair with Apple Cider Vinegar

"Glamour is about feeling good in your own skin."

—Zoe Saldana

Do you know what the most useful beauty product you can have in your home is? Is it a great skin cleanser, a toner, or a conditioner? Is it something that you apply to your skin, your hair, or your nails? There is a straightforward treatment that, believe it or not, covers all those areas and is a one-stop beauty treatment in a bottle.

It isn't even in the beauty aisle. You might even have it in your cupboard already, since it helps make a fantastic salad dressing. So, what is this mystery ingredient? It's good, old-fashioned apple cider vinegar.

You may know that ACV is beneficial for gut health and that it can help you lose weight. What you probably didn't realize is that it has also been used as a natural skin and hair care treatment since ancient times as well.

WHY IS ACV SO GOOD
TO APPLY TOPICALLY?

The most valuable benefit of ACV is that it helps to restore your skin's natural pH balance. If your skin's pH levels are not ideal, it is harder for it to look healthy and to fight off infection and bacteria. Your skin is meant to be slightly more on the acidic side to offer optimal protection and health. ACV helps your skin regain that slight acidity level that is so beneficial for it.

In addition, it contains trace elements of vitamins and minerals that your skin needs in order to stay healthy. The beta-carotene content has a substantial antioxidant effect.

The slightly astringent nature of ACV and the alpha hydroxy acids within it assist in removing dead skin cells and improving cellular turnover. So, while keeping your skin healthier, it improves its texture and radiance as well.

The malic, lactic, and acetic acids within ACV have strong antibacterial, antiseptic, and antifungal properties, making it an excellent treatment for both ridding your skin of disease and restoring it to health.

As if that wasn't enough, it also acts as an anti-inflammatory agent on inflamed skin as well. Right about now I'm sure that you are ready to dunk yourself in a whole big bathtub of the stuff. Hang on a second—that's not necessary. ACV is very useful if applied correctly. Most of the time this means diluting it. Too much of a good thing, in this case, can be bad.

I will share some recipes so that you can get the best possible beauty results for your skin and hair. Each one makes enough for one treatment, unless specified otherwise.

ACV for Your Hair

If you need to tame your locks and get frizz under control, ACV should be high on your shopping list. I advise using a raw, unfiltered variety of ACV for the best results. Don't worry about the smell—it will be strong initially but doesn't linger for very long. Here are some great recipes for you to try.

CLEAN SLATE TREATMENT

All the styling products that we use make our hair look great in the short term. The problem is that they can leave a residue that weighs the hair down and makes it look dull and lifeless. Don't waste your money on expensive clarifying shampoos, though. This simple recipe will cut right through any residue in no time. Rosemary will help reinvigorate the color of dark hair, while chamomile will help restore the shine of light hair and make it look brighter.

> 2 cups boiling water
>
> 2 teaspoons dried rosemary (for dark hair) or chamomile (for light hair)
>
> 1 cup ACV

Combine the water and herb of choice. Allow to steep for 5 minutes, remove the herb, and allow to cool. Mix 1 cup of the cooled tea with the ACV. Massage into your scalp, through to the ends of your hair. Leave in place for about 10–15 minutes, then rinse thoroughly. Add the remaining 1 cup of herbal tea to the final rinse water.

DANDRUFF TREATMENT

Just like the skin on the rest of the body, the skin of the scalp needs to be slightly more acidic in order to remain healthy. When this balance is upset on your scalp, you could end up with dry patches of skin, an itching scalp, and, embarrassingly for some people, dandruff. Use this recipe to help fight dandruff.

1 cup ACV

5 drops tea tree oil or oregano oil

5 drops lavender oil

Mix the ingredients with 1 cup of water. Massage gently into your scalp. Leave on for 10 minutes before washing your hair as usual. Your head may feel a little tingly initially, but this won't last too long.

Note: Boost this treatment by switching out the plain water for rose water (it is highly moisturizing) or rosemary, oregano, or lavender tea (each of these help to boost your hair's health and help to nourish your scalp while killing off any fungus that may be present).

DETANGLING TREATMENT

Have you decided to give up using commercial products to clean and condition your hair? You can make your own hair cleanser by using one part baking soda to three parts water. Massage this into the scalp and then into the rest of the hair. Rinse out thoroughly and then apply the following vinegar conditioning treatment.

> ½ cup ACV
>
> 3 cups herbal tea or hydrosol of your choice

Mix the ACV and tea and put it into a spray bottle. Spritz the mixture into your hair and comb through using a wide-toothed comb. Leave on for about 5 minutes and then rinse out with clean water.

Note: A hydrosol contains the essence of the herb and is not as concentrated as the tea or the essential oil. It is a good alternative if you cannot get your hands on the tea itself. Also, keep in mind that baking soda is alkaline in nature. It's best to stick to cleaning your hair with it only once or twice a week.

ANTI-FRIZZ TREATMENT

If frizzy hair plagues you, then you know that you will do almost anything to get it back under control again. The key is to keep the cuticles of the hair moisturized and smooth. Start by cleansing your hair as usual and then finishing off with a rinse made up of equal parts of ACV and water. Do the final rinse with a cold blast of water to enable the cuticles to lie flat again as they should. Use an old cotton T-shirt to dry your hair as this creates less friction than a towel does and dab your hair dry, rather than rubbing it dry. When you are ready to style your hair, use the following intensive treatment as you would a serum.

> 3 teaspoons jojoba oil (for intensive moisture)
>
> 1 teaspoon evening primrose oil (for extra nourishment)
>
> 1 teaspoon olive oil (for extra nourishment)
>
> ¼ teaspoon calendula oil (to help smooth the hair shaft)
>
> ½ teaspoon flaxseed oil (to nourish the hair)
>
> 2 drops lavender essential oil (intensively moisturizing)
>
> 2 drops saldalwood essential oil (helps to deeply moisturize)
>
> 2 drops rose essential oil (helps the hair stay hydrated)

Mix all the ingredients together well. Use only a few drops at a time, and warm it up between your hands before smoothing it over your frizzy hair. Concentrate the serum on the ends of the hair rather than just the roots.

Note: This is a great product to use if you are going to heat-style your hair. It can be applied to dry or damp hair. It can also be used as a deep-conditioning treatment as well. If you find that this serum is too intense for you in the morning, you can mix two parts of water with ACV and place it in a spritz bottle. Spritz it over the hair and style as you usually would.

Thinning Hair

Hair can start thinning for many different reasons: hormonal changes as we get older, not eating correctly, or even stress. The key is to keep the scalp as healthy as possible and to try to stimulate better circulation to your hair follicles. ACV helps to stimulate circulation and restore the health of the scalp.

TREATMENT FOR THINNING HAIR

Try this recipe if your hair is thinning for any reason.

- ½ cup ACV
- 3 cups any of the following teas: basil, hops, comfrey, peppermint, rosemary, or nettle (all help stimulate hair growth)
- 5 drops essential oil to match the herb you chose for the tea
- 5 drops lavender essential oil (intensely nourishing for the scalp and helps promote healing)

Mix together all the ingredients and massage into your scalp. The massage is as important as the ingredients because it will also help to stimulate the hair follicles. Start at the crown of your head and massage the mixture in using relatively firm circular motions, moving outward from the crown until you have covered the entire scalp. Let this massage go on for at least 5 minutes, and then, using your fingers, comb any remaining mixture through to the ends of your hair. Leave on for 5–10 minutes, and then rinse with tepid water.

Note: The scalp massage itself can stimulate extra oil production, so don't do it more than twice a week if you have oily hair. You can, however, use the recipe every day if you like; just rub it in quickly instead of massaging it in using firm strokes.

Skin Conditions

If ACV can do so much for your hair, which is mostly just dead skin cells and keratin, imagine what it can do for your living skin cells. In this section, we'll examine this further.

Psoriasis

Psoriasis normally responds very well to the application of raw ACV. ACV soothes the itch and inflammation caused by the condition. Start out carefully with ACV to make sure that the dilution is right, though. The easiest way to get relief is to add a cup of ACV to a tubful of warm, *not* hot, water and soak for at least 15 minutes.

You can also try the following recipes.

PSORIASIS BATH

Oatmeal helps to ease itching and soothe inflammation. The Epsom salt gently moisturizes the skin and nourishes it; it also aids in softening scales and alleviating itching. Rose geranium oil is one of the best oils to use to rebalance the skin, promote healing, and reduce inflammation. Lavender oil boosts the effect of the rose geranium oil, promotes healing, and reduces inflammation.

    1 cup oatmeal

    1 cup Epsom salt

    5 drops rose geranium oil

    5 drops lavender oil

    1 cup ACV

Place the oatmeal in a washcloth and secure the ends to prevent it from making a mess. Run a warm bath. While the water is running, add the washcloth with the oatmeal and the Epsom salt. Get the water to the optimal temperature and ensure that that the salts have entirely dissolved, then add the rose geranium oil, lavender oil, and ACV. Soak in the bath for at least 20 minutes, using the washcloth with the oatmeal in it to wipe down your skin.

PSORIASIS TREATMENT

Don't have time for a bath? This compress can provide almost instant relief for psoriasis itching anywhere.

> 1 cup ACV

Mix the ACV into 3 cups of tepid water in a bowl. Soak a clean washcloth in it. Wring out the cloth and apply to the affected areas. Leave it on for 2 minutes in order to get relief.

Eczema

Eczema is uncomfortable and even embarrassing for those suffering from it. It can also be challenging to treat because almost anything can set off an attack.

ACV is useful in treating the symptoms of eczema by improving the health of your skin, making it more resilient and desensitized. This makes you less prone to outbreaks in future.

In addition, ACV helps to soothe the inflammation and the itching that the attack brings on. It works in a very similar way to the treatment for psoriasis, and you can use the compress recipe detailed above to assist in dealing with an attack if you are short on time.

Need something simpler?

ECZEMA TREATMENT

The rose geranium will help to calm the irritation and promote the healing of the skin. Don't worry—the rose geranium counteracts the smell of the ACV, and the ACV smell will dissipate fairly quickly anyway.

> 1 cup ACV
>
> 1 cup rose geranium hydrosol or herbal tea

Mix the ingredients together and apply using a cotton ball. Alternatively, place in a spray bottle and spray on for larger areas. Allow the mixture to dry and go about your business as usual. This can be applied two or three times a day. Alternatively, add the entire mixture to a tubful of tepid water and soak for at least 20 minutes.

Nail Fungus

If you have ever had the misfortune of contracting a nail fungus, you will know how hard it can be to eradicate. Commercial treatments tend to be expensive and can end up causing other skin problems themselves.

ACV is ideally suited to helping you deal with this issue as well. Its antifungal properties make it one of the best options when it comes to natural treatments.

Whether you soak the affected area, use the rub, or use a combination of the two, treatment for nail fungus will take a while because it should be continued until the whole of the affected nail has grown out entirely.

Do persevere with it, though, as it is highly effective.

NAIL FUNGUS SOAK

Tea tree and oregano oil are used for their antifungal properties.

- 2 cups ACV
- 2 cups warm water
- 5 drops tea tree oil
- 5 drops oregano oil

Soak your hand or foot in the mixture for at least 30 minutes. Repeat two or three times daily until the infection is completely cleared up.

NAIL FUNGUS TREATMENT

Unfortunately, soaking your foot or hand two or three times a day is not always practical. Here's an alternative treatment. As an alternative, you can apply a few drops of the ACV directly to the nail and rub it in. Follow it up with the following mixture.

- 30 milliliters of coconut oil, melted (for its strong antifungal properties)
- 5 drops oregano oil (potent antifungal properties)
- ACV as needed

Mix the coconut oil and oregano oil. Set aside. Apply a few drops of the ACV directly to the nail and rub it in. Then rub a little of the coconut oil mixture into the nail. Repeat this three to four times a day until the infection is completely gone.

Varicose Veins

Varicose veins are unsightly, and once you have developed them, you are never going to be completely free of them. They can be a side effect of poor circulation or the weakening of the vein walls and the valves within the veins that prevent blood from flowing back into the veins instead of moving back up toward the heart.

ACV can be applied topically to help improve circulation and thus reduce the size of the veins.

VARICOSE VEIN TREATMENT

This treatment improves circulation and reduces the size of veins. In addition to this treatment, you should take other steps to improve your circulation, such as making sure that you shift position at least every 30 minutes and make attempts to be more active in general.

- ½ cup ACV
- ½ cup grapeseed oil (light and moisturizing, quickly absorbed by the skin)
- 10 drops juniper oil (boosts circulation and helps improve the tone of tissues)
- 10 drops eucalyptus oil (helps reduce inflammation and improve muscle tone)
- 10 drops sweet orange oil (helps boost circulation and improve the tone of tissues surrounding the veins)

Mix all ingredients together. Apply using gentle, upward strokes to the affected areas to stimulate circulation and reduce swelling. Use twice a day.

Deodorant

Commercial deodorants are useful, but they work by preventing you from sweating. Now, you wouldn't think that this was a bad thing because it's preventing the smell in the first place. Unfortunately, though, it is actually doing you more harm than good.

A lot of these products contain harmful ingredients, such as aluminum and agents to mask any potential smells. These can cause your pores to get blocked up, which can cause your armpits to be tender and swollen.

And it is really for nothing: It is not your sweat that causes that stale sweat smell. It is only when the bacteria naturally present on the skin break down the sweat that there is a problem with smell. So, clear off the bacteria in the area, and you can neutralize the odor.

ACV DEODORANT

Applying a paste of baking soda is a great way to neutralize the smell of sweat, but it has its own problems: After extended periods of use, your skin will start to become itchy and uncomfortable. This is because the baking soda is alkaline, and it upsets the pH balance of the skin, especially with repeated applications. How do you solve this problem? It's simple: Apply the following recipe before you use the baking soda paste, and you can kiss the stale sweat smell and irritation goodbye.

½ cup ACV

⅛ teaspoon baking soda

Mix the ACV into 1 cup of water, and place in a spray bottle. Mix the baking soda with a few drops of water to make a paste. Spray the underarm area with the ACV mixture and let it dry completely. Then, apply the baking soda paste.

Hemorrhoids

ACV assists in reducing the inflammation, itchiness, and pain that are associated with hemorrhoids and is an entirely natural treatment option.

The easiest way is by using a sitz bath. Don't get thrown by the name; it's just basically a small tub, and you can get one to fit onto your toilet. Alternatively, you might want to get a plastic basin something close to the size of a baby bath to use for this purpose. If neither option is practical, fill your regular tub to about a quarter fill, or just enough so that the water reaches the hemorrhoids.

Whichever option you use, make sure that the water is tepid rather than hot, as hot water will aggravate the symptoms. Add about 2–3 tablespoons of ACV and soak the area for about 15 minutes.

Some people advise applying straight ACV to the area as an alternative to soaking, but I advise against it, because this is a sensitive area of skin and you want to treat it gently. If you want a direct application rather than a soak, mix equal parts of ACV and water and soak a cotton ball in the mixture. You can then dab on as required two or three times a day.

Burns

The primary problem when it comes to burned skin is that it can become infected very quickly. The recipe provided below can help to prevent infection and assist in the healing process. There is a strong cautionary note here, however: You must only use this for minor burns and *only* in this diluted form. Straight ACV, in this case, is going to do more harm than good.

BURN TREATMENT

Straight lavender oil can be applied to the skin, and so it is being included here. It is especially effective at promoting the healing of burns and reducing the incidence of scarring.

½ cup ACV

10 drops lavender oil

Mix the ACV and lavender oil into 1 cup of water. Place in a sprayer and spray onto the burn, or apply using a cotton ball.

Note: *Never* use this treatment with severe burns. Get medical help for those.

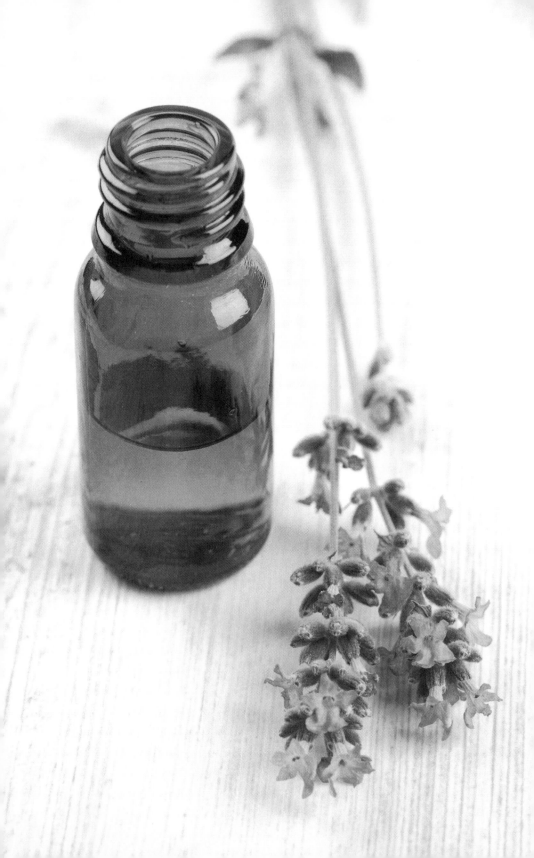

Sunburn

ACV can help remove the sting from sunburn, reduce inflammation, and help prevent your skin from blistering. It also promotes healing.

SUNBURN TREATMENT

Lavender, rose geranium, and palma rosa oil are used for their ability to regenerate and heal the skin. Together these three make a potent skin healing mixture that will give the skin the extra nourishment that it needs at this time.

> 1 cup ACV
>
> 10 drops lavender oil
>
> 5 drops rose geranium oil
>
> 5 drops palma rosa oil

Mix the ACV and oils with 4 cups of cold water in a bowl. Soak a clean washcloth in the mixture. Wring it out and apply as a cold compress to the affected areas. Follow up by applying some aloe vera gel to complete the healing process.

Alternative: Add the ACV and the essential oils to a tepid bath of water and soak for 20–25 minutes. It may sting a little initially, but it won't for long.

Sunspots

We may love the sun, but it is not so great for our skin, even when it doesn't burn us. As we get older, we are more prone to developing sunspots. The best cure for these is to try to prevent them from forming in the first place. This means taking measures to protect yourself from the sun when you are out and about.

That's not always practical, though, and sometimes, no matter how careful you are, they might still develop. Fortunately, the alpha hydroxy acids present in ACV can help to minimize the appearance of these marks by removing the upper layer of dead skin cells and promoting the development of a healthier underlying layer.

SUNSPOT TREATMENT 1

Neroli oil and rose oil are nourishing for mature or damaged skin and promote cell turnover. Rose oil, in addition, can help to even out differences in skin tone. Rose hip oil is used as a base because it, too, is excellent for dry and damaged skin and can help protect the skin against further sun damage. It is very rich and great as part of a night treatment product.

    ½ cup ACV
    1 cup rose hip oil
    5 drops neroli essential oil
    5 drops rose essential oil

Mix all ingredients together and apply to sunspots at night before going to bed.

Note: This mixture should *not* be used if you are about to go out into the sun because the neroli oil is phototoxic. This means that it will react with UV radiation and cause skin irritation and darkening. If you stick to using it only at night, you'll be fine.

SUNSPOT TREATMENT 2

If you want something lighter that is also suitable for daytime use, try this recipe. Honey is a humectant that helps lock moisture into the skin. It is also highly nourishing.

½ cup ACV

½ cup raw honey

5 drops of rose essential oil

Mix the ACV, honey, and rose essential oil together with 1 cup of water. Apply to the affected area. Leave it to soak in for about 15 minutes, then rinse off any residue with warm water.

Bruises

ACV can be applied to bruised skin to help reduce the inflammation, improve circulation, and help the bruise fade faster.

BRUISE TREATMENT

This recipe will sort out bruising fast. Use this as soon as possible after the injury, and you may even be able to prevent a bad bruise from developing. If you are already bruised, do this twice a day, and your bruise will clear up in no time.

> ½ cup ACV
>
> Arnica oil

Mix the ACV into 1 cup of water. Soak a clean washcloth in the mixture, wring it out, and apply as a cold compress to the affected area. Leave in place for 15–20 minutes. Remove the cloth and allow the area to dry naturally. Then apply enough Arnica oil to cover the bruise. Leave it to be absorbed.

Pimples and Acne

The problem with over-the-counter acne treatments is that, while they may clear up the acne quickly, they are very harsh on the underlying skin. This could leave your skin feeling dry and uncomfortable and more prone to breakouts in the future as the skin starts increasing sebum output to compensate.

ACV scores big points in this department because it not only clears up the bacteria that cause inflammation, it also helps reduce inflammation and restores the skin's natural pH levels.

Your skin is better able to regulate itself, so sebum levels go back to normal. The astringent nature of the ACV helps to clear dead skin cells and keep the pores clear. The result is clearer skin that is healthier and less prone to breakouts.

ACNE TREATMENT

You can choose to use a hydrosol or herbal tea in place of the water to boost the skin-healing properties. Choose which herb to use based on the skin type of the underlying skin. If you have dry skin that is acne-prone, use a gentle herb such as chamomile or rose. If you have oilier skin that is acne-prone, choose an herb such as rosemary or lemon balm.

½ cup ACV

Mix the ACV into 1 cup of water or tea and apply to the skin. Leave it on for about 10 minutes, and then rinse it off. Follow with your regular moisturizing routine.

PIMPLE SPOT TREATMENT

If you don't have a problem with acne, but just get an occasional pimple, ACV can act as an excellent spot treatment. Tea tree oil will kill off any bacteria that could cause infection. The antibacterial properties of the ACV are equally useful, but this combination delivers a one-two punch that no pimple can stand up against. ACV is also helpful in reducing inflammation and promoting healing in the area.

> ½ cup ACV
>
> 2 drops tea tree oil

Mix the ACV and tea tree oil into ½ cup of water. Apply the mixture as soon as you see a pimple coming up, and it will prevent it from forming an ugly head. **Note:** If you want a low-cost, efficient toner for your skin, just omit the tea tree oil and double the water content. Apply with a cotton ball to remove any last traces of cleanser and debris and to tone the pores of your skin. Follow as usual with your moisturizer.

Face Masks for Different Skin Types

ACV can also be incorporated into your weekly skin care routine by including it in your face masks. Just choose the right ingredients for your skin type.

DRY SKIN FACE MASK

I am cheating a little here. This mask does not contain ACV. But before you use it, clean your skin and then exfoliate it with ACV diluted in a 1:3 ratio with plain water. Rinse, and then apply the mask.

- ¼ cup unscented aqueous cream or lotion of your choice
- 1 cup kaolin clay (helps to draw out impurities without being overharsh on the skin)
- ½ cup oatmeal, ground very finely
- ½ cup raw honey
- 5 drops palma rosa essential oil
- 5 drops rose geranium essential oil
- 5 drops lavender oil

Blend all ingredients together, and apply to your face, avoiding your eye area. Sit back and relax for 15 minutes, then rinse off the mask with tepid water.

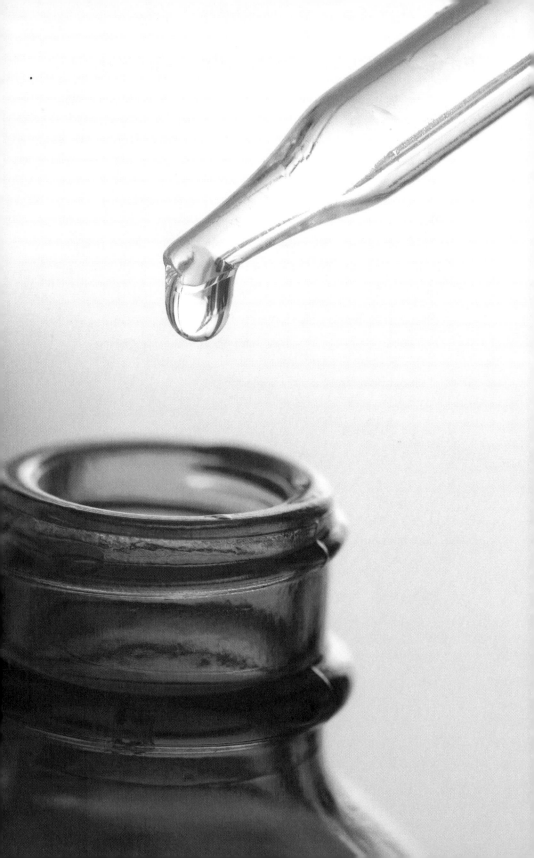

OILY SKIN FACE MASK

Many recipes for oily skin include witch hazel as an astringent. ACV is just as effective and kinder on your skin.

    ½ cup kaolin clay

    ½ cup activated charcoal (helps to draw out impurities)

    1 tablespoon raw honey (helps clear bacteria and keep skin moist)

    2 teaspoons ACV

    ½ cup glycerin

    4 drops cypress essential oil

    2 drops juniper essential oil

    5 drops eucalyptus essential oil

Blend all ingredients together, and apply to your face. Leave on for at least 20 minutes, then rinse off using tepid water.

SENSUOUS FACIAL TONING SPRAY

Makes enough for 30 uses

        5 ounces water

        1 ounce witch hazel

        1 tablespoon ACV

        5 drops sandalwood essential oil

        3 drops cedarwood essential oil

        5 drops rose essential oil

Pour all ingredients into a spray bottle. Close, then shake vigorously.

ACV ROSE HIP LUSCIOUS FACIAL TREATMENT

⅛ cup rose hip oil

⅛ cup jojoba oil

1 drop rose oil

3 cups water

1 tablespoon ACV

Combine the three oils and massage them into your face starting from the center of the face and working out in small circles to promote lymphatic gland drainage in the face. Do this for 3 to 5 minutes. Remove with a warm cloth. Then combine the water and apple cider vinegar and splash face to tone. This treatment is best done before bedtime.

Cellulite

When it comes to cellulite, the problem is not so much that it exists, but the lack of tone of the skin tissue on top of it. While cellulite can be hard to shift, ACV can go a long way to restoring the tone of the skin and to improving circulation.

CELLULITE TREATMENT

This mixture draws in the moisturizing properties of either coconut oil or olive oil to help smooth out the skin. For this purpose, I prefer coconut oil; it is semisolid at room temperature and thus less messy to apply. I also like the smell. In addition, the lauric acid in it has better skin toning and smoothing properties than olive oil does. However, coconut oil can cause rashes in some individuals when used over an extended period, so you need to watch out for that. The essential oils jump-start circulation and help to further tone the skin. Just keep in mind that sweet orange oil is phototoxic, so avoid sun exposure after applying the mixture. If you are concerned about this, it can be safely left out.

> 1 cup coconut or olive oil (you may need to melt the coconut oil a little)
>
> 3 cups ACV
>
> 25 drops sweet orange oil
>
> 25 drops juniper oil

Mix all ingredients together well. Apply to the affected areas in the morning and evening.

Soothing Razor Burn

The idea of applying vinegar to freshly shaved skin is not appealing. It will sting. That is not what I am telling you to do here. Use a mixture of half ACV and half water to the area the following day. This helps to soothe irritation and inflammation and prevent the area from getting infected. It will also help prevent ingrown hairs by exfoliating the skin gently.

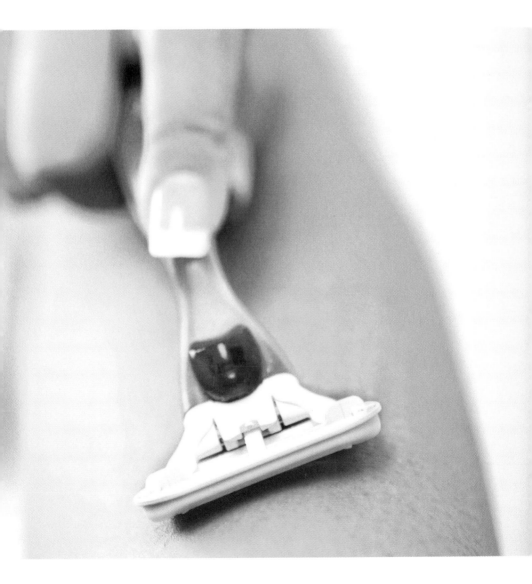

Other Health and Beauty Uses for ACV

RELAXING LINEN SPRAY

Makes enough for 30 uses

    5½ ounces water

    1 tablespoon ACV

    5 drops lavender essential oil

    5 drops Roman chamomile essential oil

Pour all ingredients into a spray bottle. Close, then shake vigorously.

ACV BLISSFUL ROSE BATH

    1 cup ACV

    1 cup Epsom salt

    1 cup dried rose petals

Run a hot bath and add all ingredients. Mix and soak.

ACV TRANQUIL CHAMOMILE BATH

1 cup ACV

1 cup Epsom salt

1 cup dried chamomile

Run a hot bath and add all ingredients. Mix and soak.

ACV REFRESHING MINT BATH

1 cup ACV

1 cup Epsom salt

1 cup fresh mint leaves

1 drop spearmint essential oil

Run a hot bath and add all ingredients. Mix and soak.

ACV LAVENDER BODY POLISH

   1 cup coarse sea salt

   ½ cup coconut oil

   ½ cup ACV

   ¼ cup dried lavender

Combine all ingredients with a wooden spoon in a bowl. Use as scrub in the shower and rinse thoroughly after use.

ENLIVENING AIR FRESHENING SPRAY

Makes enough for 30 uses

   5½ ounces water

   1 tablespoon ACV

   5 drops lime essential oil

   5 drops lemongrass essential oil

   5 drops bergamot essential oil

Pour all ingredients into a 6-ounce spray bottle. Close, and shake vigorously.

FRUIT AND VEGGIE WASH

Makes enough for 30 uses

    4½ ounces water

    1 ounce ACV

    2 drops lemon essential oil

Pour all ingredients into a spray bottle. Close, then shake vigorously. Spray whole produce thoroughly. Rinse. Enjoy.

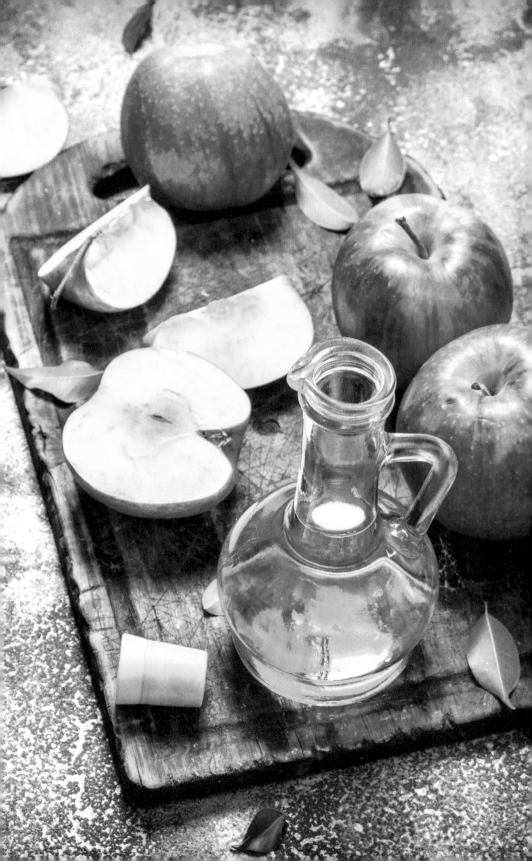

Chapter 12

Scrumptious Apple Cider Vinegar Recipes

"You don't have to cook fancy or complicated master-pieces—just good food from fresh ingredients."

—Julia Child

Cooking with apple cider vinegar provides a tremendous opportunity to add health-boosting power to your diet while not scrimping on flavor. Apple cider vinegar has a delicious, distinctive flavor that you can enjoy in a variety of dishes and preparations. It can be used for its medicinal properties but also for its ability to flavor recipes with its unique, distinctive effervescence. Because it is a fermented liquid, it offers extra-powerful nutritional value. It contains prebiotic and probiotic compounds that can restore your health in gentle and subtle ways that can be felt long term. That's why long-term consumption of apple cider vinegar is even better than short-term because you will be supporting your health on a regular basis in an easy-to-sustain manner. So, add apple cider vinegar to your cooking regimen today!

The recipes in this chapter were chosen because they are extremely tasty and extremely healthy. All the recipes make use of one wonder ingredient in particular: ACV.

Organic, unfiltered ACV is a powerhouse of nutrients and prebiotic compounds that help the beneficial gut bacteria to regain the upper hand. Your energy levels and health will improve, and you'll feel a lot more vital again.

Appetizers

BASIL-ZUCCHINI BRUSCHETTA

Serves 4

   3 zucchini, chopped

   1 cup watercress, chopped

   1 avocado, cubed

   1 bunch fresh basil, chopped

   ½ teaspoon ACV

   1 tablepoon avocado oil

   Dash cracked pepper

   Toast points or pita squares (for serving)

Stir ingredients together and serve on toast points or pita squares.

HALLOUMI BRUSCHETTA

Serves 4

    1 baguette

    7 ounces halloumi

    2 tablespoons ACV

    1 tablespoon honey

    3 Roma tomatoes, thinly sliced and deseeded

    1 bunch fresh basil leaves

    Fresh cracked pepper, to taste

Slice baguette, place on a baking sheet, and broil for 2 minutes until golden brown. Remove from oven and cover. Slightly preheat a nonstick frying pan. Slice halloumi into ¼-inch slices and place in pan. Cook both sides until golden brown, turning once. Heat apple cider vinegar and honey in a small saucepan on medium heat for 5 minutes. Stir continually. Arrange baguette slices on a serving dish. Place one piece of halloumi on each slice. Drizzle apple cider vinegar glaze over cheese. Top with a slice of Roma tomato and a fresh basil leaf. Season to taste with fresh cracked pepper.

Soups

BLACK BEAN STEW AND BROWN RICE

Serves 4

1 tablespoon extra virgin olive oil

1 garlic clove, finely chopped

1 medium mild onion, finely chopped

Salt and pepper, to taste

2½ cans (about 38 ounces) black beans, rinsed and drained

1 tablespoon ACV

½ teaspoon dried oregano

1 can (14½ ounces) vegetable broth

1½ cups brown rice, cooked and drained

Heat the oil in a large saucepan over medium-high heat. Add the garlic and onion to the pan, and season with pepper. Fry, stirring often until the onion is soft. Add the beans, ACV, oregano, and broth, and season with salt and additional pepper, if needed. Cook for about 7 minutes, and then serve with the rice.

TURMERIC AND GINGER SOUP

Serves 4

Turmeric is nature's prime anti-inflammatory agent. In studies, curcumin, the active ingredient in turmeric, has been shown to be as effective as some commercial anti-inflammatories. The ginger in this soup adds more than just some zing; it is also a very effective anti-inflammatory and bolsters the digestive process. The garlic has potent antioxidant effects.

1 tablespoon coconut oil

1 large onion, finely sliced

2 stalks celery, finely sliced

1 carrot, finely sliced

1 teaspoon powdered turmeric

3 or 4 cloves of garlic, finely sliced

6 cups vegetable broth

Salt and pepper, to taste

2 cups cauliflower, finely sliced

1 tablespoon fresh ginger, peeled and finely sliced

2 cups kale, finely sliced

1 teaspoon ACV

1 can (15 ounces) garbanzo beans, rinsed and drained

Melt the coconut oil in a large saucepan over medium-low heat. Stir in the onion, and cook until it begins to br own. Add the celery and carrots, and cook for a few minutes until softened. Stir in the turmeric and garlic, and make sure that the veggies are as evenly coated as possible. Cook for 1 minute before adding the broth, salt, and pepper. Allow the soup to come to a boil, stirring often. Add the cauliflower and ginger and reduce the heat to low. Cover and allow the soup to cook until the cauliflower is cooked through, about 10 minutes. Add the kale, ACV, and beans, and cover. Cook for another few minutes until the kale wilts.

Salads & Main Coures

ACV SALAD DRESSING

Serves 4

Incorporate the immune-boosting benefits of both ACV and honey. Olive oil adds fat.

> 1 spring onion, cleaned and chopped
>
> ⅓ cup extra virgin olive oil
>
> 2 teaspoons mild mustard
>
> ¼ cup ACV
>
> 2 teaspoons honey
>
> ½ teaspoon coriander
>
> Salt and pepper, to taste

Blend all ingredients together until they form a smooth paste. If needed, add a little more olive oil and ACV to get your preferred consistency. The dressing will keep for 6–7 days in the refrigerator.

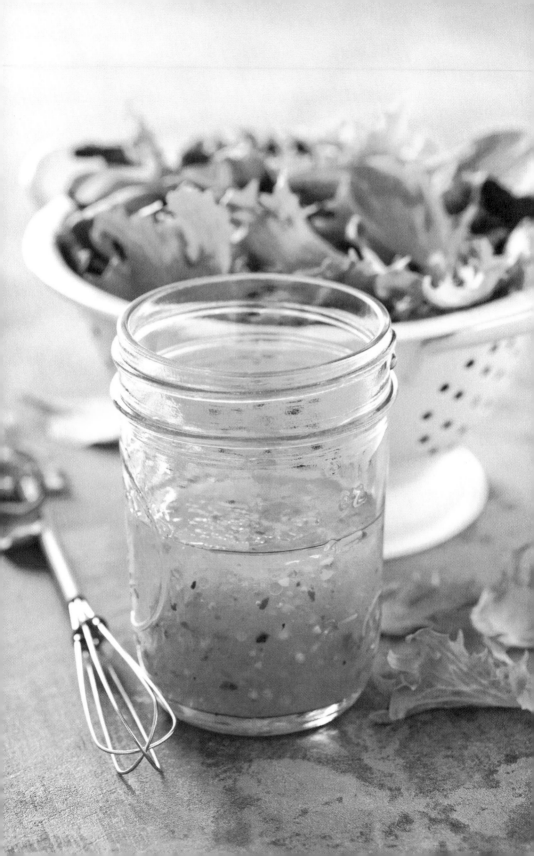

QUINOA AND PLUMS WITH ACV DRESSING

Serves 4

The quinoa in this dish gives a healthy dash of protein. The fresh green beans add fiber and nutrients. The plums are packed with vitamins and give a satisfying crunch to the meal. The olive oil and pecan nuts provide good fats for your body.

FOR THE QUINOA:

- ½ cup raw quinoa
- Enough vegetable stock to completely cover the quinoa

FOR THE DRESSING:

- ¼ cup olive oil
- 1 teaspoon mustard
- ½ cup ACV
- 2 tablespoons honey
- Salt, to taste

FOR THE GREEN BEANS:

- 2 tablespoons olive oil
- 4 cloves garlic, minced
- 16 ounces green beans, cleaned and chopped into 1-inch pieces
- ½ teaspoon dried dill
- Salt and pepper, to taste

FOR THE SALAD:

- 5 ounces arugula or baby kale
- 4 ounces mild goat cheese, crumbled
- 2 plums, cored and cubed
- Pecans, coarsely chopped, to taste

Prepare the quinoa: Make the quinoa as directed on the package, using vegetable stock instead of water. Cover and set aside.

Prepare the dressing: Mix together the dressing ingredients.

Prepare the green beans: Heat the olive oil in a frying pan over medium heat. Add the garlic, green beans, and dill, and season with salt and pepper. Cook about 2 minutes; the beans should still be firm.

Assemble the salad: When you're ready to serve, arrange the arugula on plates, then add the quinoa. Top with the goat cheese. Layer the green beans and plums on top. Sprinkle with pecans, and drizzle on the dressing.

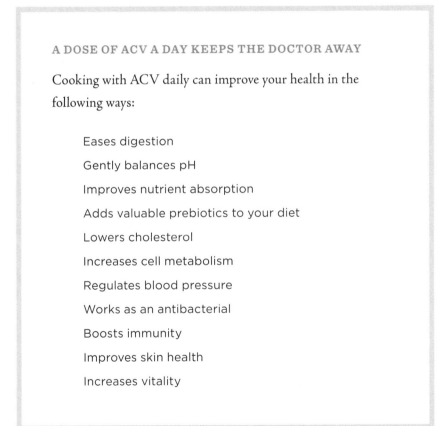

A DOSE OF ACV A DAY KEEPS THE DOCTOR AWAY

Cooking with ACV daily can improve your health in the following ways:

Eases digestion

Gently balances pH

Improves nutrient absorption

Adds valuable prebiotics to your diet

Lowers cholesterol

Increases cell metabolism

Regulates blood pressure

Works as an antibacterial

Boosts immunity

Improves skin health

Increases vitality

KALE AND AVOCADO SALAD

Serves 2

 1 bunch kale, ribs removed

 1 tablespoon olive oil

 ¼ cup ACV

 Juice of ½ lemon

 Salt, to taste

 1 avocado, diced

 8 ounces cherry tomatoes, cut in half

 ¼ cup sunflower seeds

 ¼ cup finely diced mild onion

Chop the kale into manageable pieces and put it on a serving dish.
Mix together the olive oil, ACV, lemon juice, and salt until completely
incorporated. Pour over the kale and rub into the pieces so that they soften.
Top with the remaining ingredients and serve.

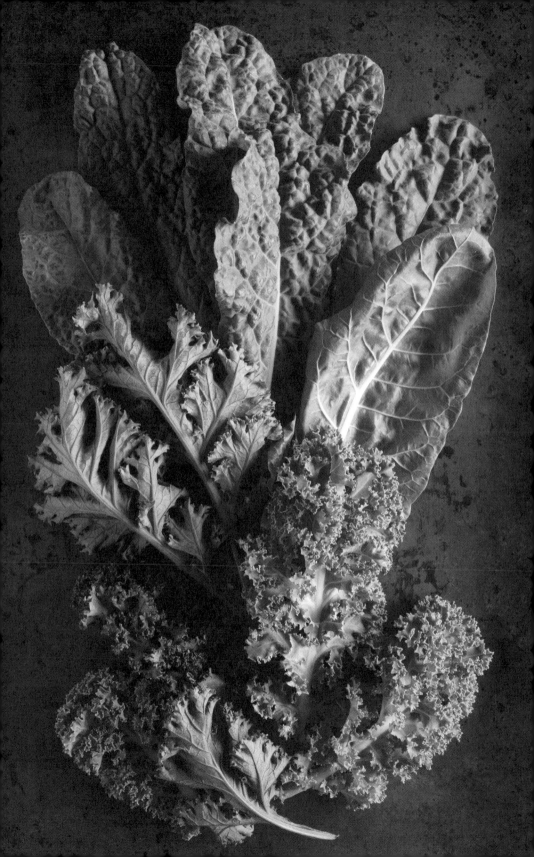

FRUITY ACV SALAD

Serves 4

The wheat berries and beans in this recipe provide valuable nutrients and fiber. The peaches and strawberries lend a nice sweet flavor to the meal and also come with a lot of fiber and nutrients. The blueberries are packed with antioxidants. Kale is one of nature's most versatile superfoods, brimming with antioxidants and immune-boosting nutrients. The almonds and olive oil provide healthy fats and important nutrients. The cinnamon has a balancing effect on blood sugar levels.

1 cup raw wheat berries

15 ounces canned garbanzo beans, drained and rinsed

5 cups raw kale, chopped

3 tablespoons olive oil, divided

2 cups peaches, finely chopped

1 cup blueberries

1 cup strawberries, finely sliced

½ cup almonds, finely chopped

Cinnamon, to taste

¼ cup ACV

2 tablespoons pure maple syrup

1 teaspoon Dijon mustard

Salt, to taste

In a large pot, combine 3 cups of water with the wheat berries. Bring to a boil and cook over medium-high heat for approximately 30 minutes, or until the berries are tender. Drain well, and then stir in the beans. Set aside. Fry the kale with 2 teaspoons of the olive oil in a large skillet over medium-high heat until it is tender. Mix the kale into the beans and wheat berries. Mix in the peaches, blueberries, strawberries, almonds, and cinnamon. In a separate bowl, combine the ACV, maple syrup, the remaining 1 tablespoon of olive oil, mustard, and salt, and pour over the wheat berry mixture. \

SEAWEED SALAD

Serves 4

> 1 ounce dehydrated seaweed or kelp noodles
>
> 1 tablespoon ACV
>
> 1 tablespoon sesame oil
>
> ½ teaspoon minced ginger
>
> 1 tablespoon soy sauce
>
> Salt, to taste
>
> 1 scallion, finely chopped
>
> 1 tablespoon toasted sesame seeds

Fill a bowl with chilled water and let the seaweed soak for 5 minutes. In the meantime, mix all remaining ingredients together. Drain the seaweed, and squeeze out as much water as you can. Serve with the dressing.

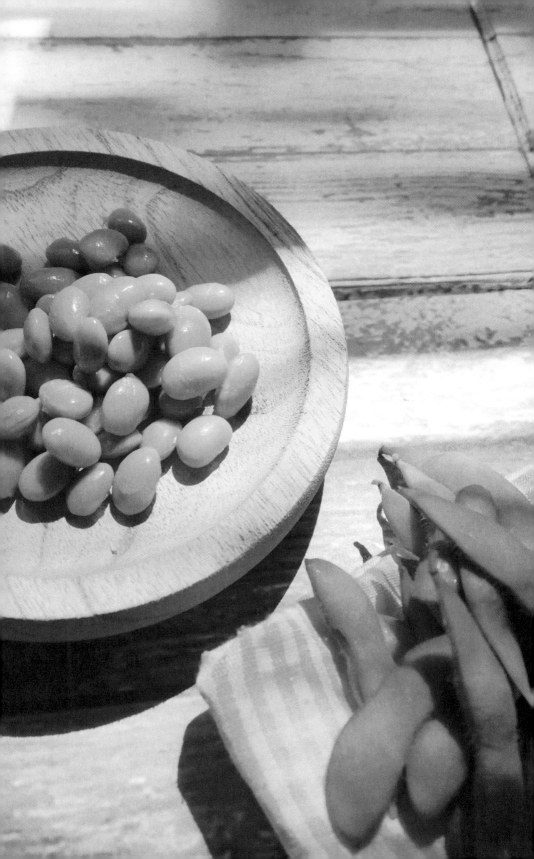

EDAMAME SALAD

Serves 4

    1 pound shelled edamame

    1 pound green peas

    12 ounces black soybeans, rinsed and drained

    ½ onion, finely sliced

    ¼ cup olive oil

    ¼ cup ACV

    Salt and pepper, to taste

    ½ bunch fresh basil, chopped

Mix together all the ingredients. Refrigerate for 30 minutes to allow flavors to develop.

PARSLEY BLACK-RICE SALAD

Serves 4

Parsley is packed with nutrients and good for helping to clear toxins from the body. The cucumber and lemon provide valuable nutrients and a healthy dose of fiber. The onion and garlic help to boost immunity and fight off colds and flu. The mint will help to soothe digestive issues. The black rice provides a huge nutrient punch and also provides fiber that is essential for good gut health.

> 1 stalk spring onion, finely chopped
>
> Paprika, to taste
>
> Cumin, to taste
>
> Salt, to taste
>
> 3 cups black rice
>
> 2 cups parsley, finely chopped
>
> 1 cucumber, skinned and finely chopped
>
> 1 clove garlic, minced
>
> Mint leaves, finely chopped, to taste
>
> Dash olive oil
>
> Juice of ½ lemon
>
> ½ teaspoon ACV

Mix the spring onion with the paprika, cumin, and salt. Cook the rice according to the directions on the package. Mix the rice with the onion mixture and the remaining ingredients, and serve immediately.

SPINACH WITH QUINOA AND CHICKPEAS

Serves 4

Spinach has lots of beneficial chlorophyll and minerals.

- 3 tablespoons olive oil
- 1 tablespoon ACV
- 1 tablespoon raw honey
- 1 teaspoon mustard powder
- 1 cup baby spinach
- ½ cup cooked quinoa
- ½ cup cooked chickpeas
- ½ cup cooked artichoke hearts
- 8 cherry tomatoes
- ½ avocado, peeled and cubed

Mix together the olive oil, ACV, honey, and mustard powder until completely incorporated and set aside. Mix together the remaining ingredients, and top with the apple cider vinegar mixture just before serving.

VEGAN ACV "SUSHI"

Serves 2

> 1 cup rice
>
> 1 tablespoon ACV
>
> 1 tablespoon sugar
>
> Salt, to taste

FILLINGS:

> Choose from thinly sliced carrot sticks, thinly sliced cucumbers
> sticks, mung bean sprouts, fresh mint leaves, fresh cilantro,
> fresh basil, green beans, arugula stalks, leeks sliced lengthwise,
> apples sliced into sticks
>
> Black sesame seeds

Put the rice into a bowl and cover with water. Stir well until the water starts to get cloudy. Strain the rice and repeat until the water is clear. Put the rice in a pot and add 2 cups of water. Bring the mixture to a boil over medium-high heat. Lower the heat and put the lid on the pot. Simmer for 15 minutes, or until the water is completely absorbed. Remove from the heat and stir quickly. Put the lid back on and set aside. In the meantime, mix together the ACV, sugar, and salt, and heat gently in a small saucepan for a few minutes. Gently mix the ACV mixture into the rice. Form the rice mixture into a sheet, place your chosen ingredients in the center, and roll it up using a sushi mat. These are often made of bamboo and you can find them at your favorite cooking supply store. Feel free to layer an optional sheet of nori seaweed on top of the rice and under the filling if you would like. Sprinkle the veggie sushi with black sesame seeds, and then slice the roll into pieces.

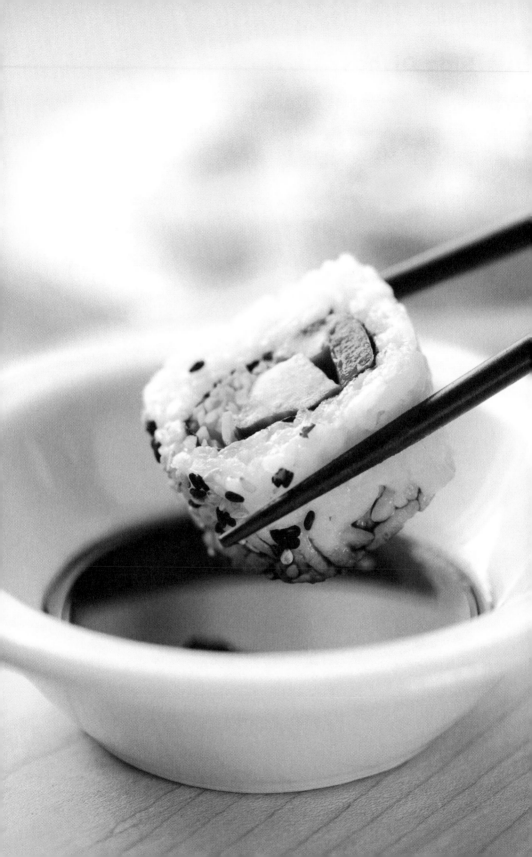

Side Dishes

BLACK BEAN LOW ACID SALSA

Serves 4

    1 can black beans, drained

    ½ cup chopped onion

    ½ cup chopped cilantro

    2 cubed avocados

    ½ cup fresh pineapple, chopped (optional)

    1 teaspoon ACV

    1 teaspoon lime juice

    ½ teaspoon Celtic sea salt

    ¼ teaspoon chili powder

    ¼ teaspoon paprika

    Corn or white bean chips (for serving)

Stir all ingredients together and serve with corn or white bean chips.

GUACAMOLE

Serves 4

Avocados are packed with healthy fats and nutrients.

- 2 avocados, pitted, peeled, and cubed
- 2 tablespoons ACV
- 1 teaspoon dried chives
- 2 tablespoons fresh lime juice
- Salt and pepper, to taste
- ¼ cup fresh cilantro, coarsely chopped
- ½ Roma tomato, chopped finely

Combine the avocados, ACV, chives, lime juice, salt, and pepper in a blender. Remove the mixture from the blender, and stir in the cilantro and tomatoes. Serve immediately.

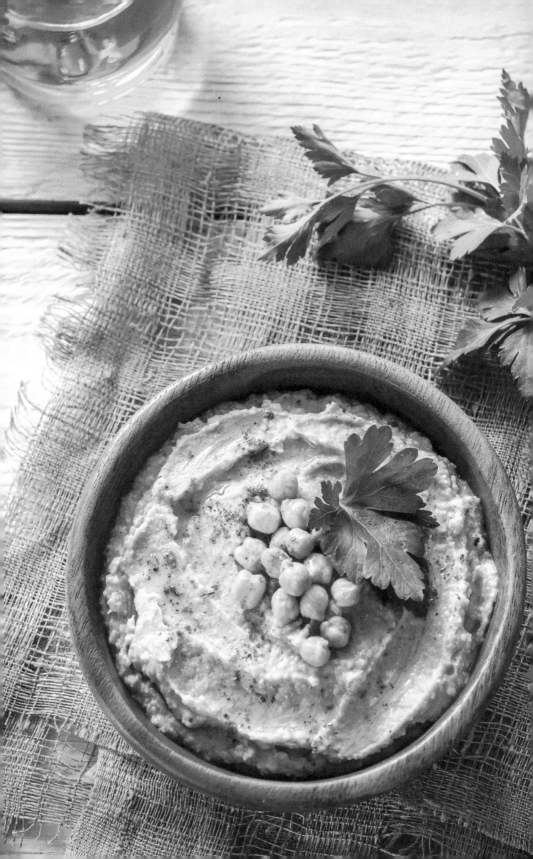

HUMMUS

Serves 4

Chickpeas are high in protein. The tahini gives you a dose of healthy fat.

- ¼ cup olive oil
- 15 ounces canned chickpeas, rinsed and drained
- 3 garlic cloves
- 2 tablespoons tahini
- 3 tablespoons fresh lemon juice
- 2 teaspoons cumin
- 1 tablespoon ACV
- Salt, to taste
- ½ teaspoon paprika

Combine all ingredients with 2 tablespoons of water in a blender and blend until smooth.

CANNED PICKLED APPLES

Yields about 7 pints

If you are a fan of making jams you will love this canning recipe!

- 4 cups ACV
- 6 cups sugar
- 4 cinnamon sticks, lightly crushed
- 2 tablespoons whole cloves
- 8 pounds apples, peeled, chopped, and cored

Mix the ACV and sugar with 2 cups of water in a big pot. Place the cinnamon and cloves in a small muslin bag so that you can fish them out easily after cooking. Bring the mixture to a boil over medium-high heat. Boil, stirring often, until all the sugar has dissolved. Add the apples and cook for another 30 minutes, or until the apples soften. Refrigerate for at least 24 hours before canning the apples to allow the flavors to develop. Fill sterilized canning jars with the apples, leaving room for the syrup. Remove the muslin bag from of the syrup, and bring the syrup to a boil again. Divide the syrup up among the jars of apples. Seal as usual.

Drinks

CRANBERRY ACV SPRITZ

Serves 2

The cranberry juice is packed with antioxidants.

 ¼ cup ACV

 ¼ cup cranberry juice

 3 cups sparkling water

 4 teaspoons maple syrup

Mix all ingredients together.

ACV ENERGY BOOST

Serves 1

Molasses is jam-packed with vitamins and minerals necessary for great health.

 2 tablespoons ACV

 2 teaspoons blackstrap molasses

Stir the ingredients into 1½ cups of plain water.

ACV VIRGIN MARY

Serves 1

1½ cups tomato juice

2 tablespoons ACV

Pinch salt

Hot sauce, to taste

Stir all the ingredients together.

ACV GRAPEFRUIT COOLER

Serves 1

The grapefruit juice is high in antioxidants and promotes weight loss.

1½ cups freshly squeezed grapefruit juice

2 tablespoons ACV

2 tablespoons raw honey

Mix all the ingredients together.

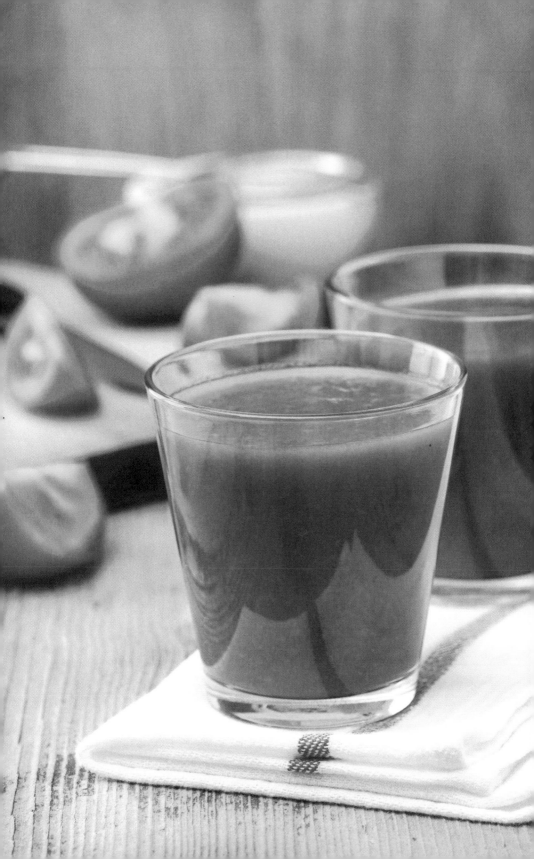

Desserts

APPLE CHOCOLATE ALMOND BUTTER BALLS

Serves 6

3 cups almond butter

3 cups shredded coconut (unsweetened)

½ cup chia seeds

¼ maple syrup

¼ cup apple, chopped very finely (not peeled)

½ teaspoon ACV

1 cup raw dark chocolate, chopped (lightly sweetened or unsweetened)

Mix all ingredients except chocolate with a wooden spoon. Chill for 15 minutes then form into balls. Coat with chocolate by rolling balls gently after forming. Store layered in parchment paper in a sealed container, and place the container in the refrigerator.

APPLE BANANA SORBET

Serves 2

6 frozen bananas, peeled and sliced

1 frozen apple, peeled and chopped

¼ teaspoon ACV

Apple juice or water (optional)

Dash powdered cinnamon

Add all ingredients except cinnamon to blender and mix on high until smooth. You can add a little bit of apple juice or water as needed to help the ingredients blend but you want to use the smallest amount of liquid possible to retain the sorbet's texture. Garnish with powdered cinnamon.

BERRY BLAST FOR SHORTCAKE

Serves 4

    1 cup sliced fresh strawberries

    1 cup fresh blueberries

    1 cup fresh blackberries

    1 cup fresh raspberries

    ½ cup fresh red or black currants

    2 tablespoons ACV

    1 tablespoon sugar

    Shortcake (for serving)

    Whipped cream (for serving)

    ½ cup fresh mint leaves (for garnish)

Mix all ingredients, except for the last three, and store in a sealed container in the refrigerator overnight. Serve over shortcake and top with whipped cream. Garnish with mint leaves.

MINTY-GREEN ICE POPS

Serves 4

    4 cups frozen green grapes

    1 frozen kiwi, peeled and chopped

    1 large bunch mint

    ¼ teaspoon ACV

    Water or green tea (optional)

Blend all ingredients in a blender on high until smooth. You can add a little water or green tea as needed to create the desired texture. Then pour mixture into ice-pop molds, freeze, and enjoy.

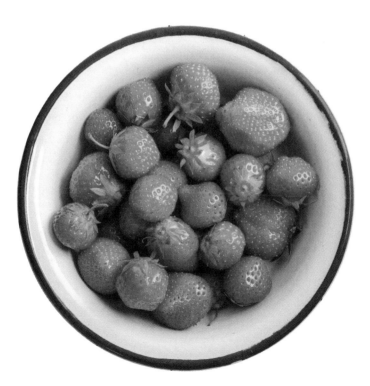

VEGAN BLUEBERRY CAKE

Serves 4

¾ cup sugar

1¾ cups flour

¼ teaspoon salt

¼ cup cocoa powder

1 teaspoon baking soda

⅓ cup melted coconut oil

1 cup plain water

1 teaspoon ACV

1 teaspoon vanilla extract

1 cup blueberries

Preheat the oven to 350°F. Grease a standard-sized loaf pan. Mix together the sugar, flour, salt, cocoa powder, and baking soda. In a separate bowl, mix together the coconut oil, water, ACV, and vanilla. Fold the dry ingredients into the wet ingredients, and mix until they are fully incorporated. Gently fold in the blueberries. Put the batter into the loaf pan. Bake in the center of the oven for 40 minutes, or until a toothpick inserted in the center comes out clean.

ACV CARAMEL SAUCE FOR ICE CREAM

Yields 2 cups

This is a really delicious way to get some ACV into your diet.

2 cups apple cider

1 tablespoon ACV

¾ cup granulated sugar

¼ cup light brown sugar

½ cup heavy cream

2 tablespoons butter

Pinch ground cinnamon

Pinch salt

½ teaspoon vanilla extract

Combine the apple cider and ACV in a large pot over medium-high heat. Bring it to a boil, stirring occasionally. Once it boils, stir frequently for another 10–15 minutes, until the sauce is reduced to about ½ cup and becomes very thick. Lower the heat to medium-low and add the granulated sugar and brown sugar. Let the mixture come to a slow boil, stirring all the while until the sugar has dissolved completely. Add the cream and butter. Bring this mixture to a boil, stirring continuously, until the mixtures thickens a bit. Remove from the heat and add the cinnamon, salt, and vanilla. Allow to cool and thicken, and serve over ice cream.

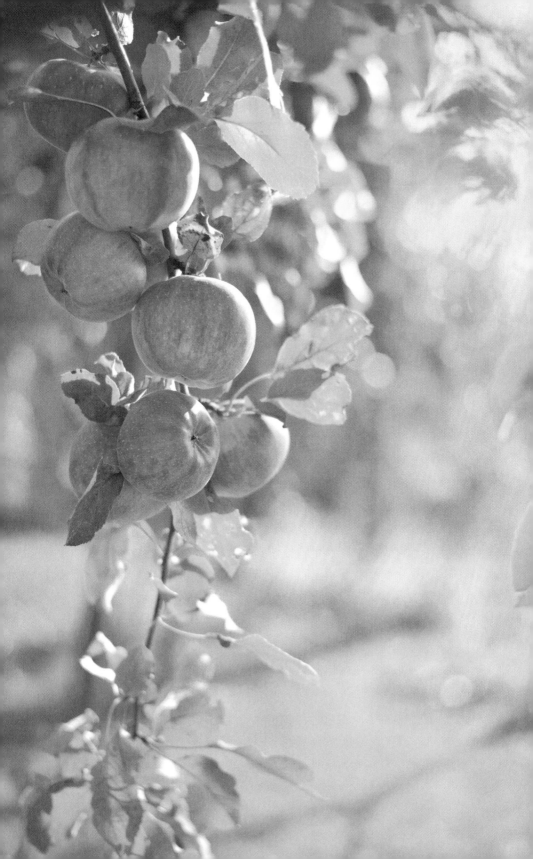

Chapter 13

Frequently Asked Questions

Okay, so what is ACV?

ACV is a sour liquid derived from apples. It is commonly used as a remedy for various ailments, as a health booster, and even as a cleaning product. The stories and folklore around ACV are just the beginning of the exciting benefits associated with this elixir.

How much ACV is helpful and safe to consume in one day?

Everyone knows that one person who always takes things a little too far. Maybe that person is you. ACV boasts health benefits, but, like all things, should be consumed in moderation. Currently, health professionals do not agree on an exact amount of ACV to consume a day, but general consensus points to a daily intake of 1 tablespoon with a glass of water. Because this aspect of ACV is unknown and variable by each person, speak with your doctor to see if ACV is safe for you in any amount.

Is it better to consume ACV with the mother?

The mother (also sometimes called the SCOBY) is simply the enzymes, proteins, and bacteria that give ACV its benefits. Even though it looks like a sludgy cobweb trapped in the bottle, it is good that it is there. This type of ACV is known as unrefined and unfiltered and has not gone through the process of pasteurization. Consuming ACV with the mother gives you more of the beneficial bacteria—key items that are removed during the pasteurization process.

Is ACV still healthy to consume when it is cooked?

ACV is a great addition to the kitchen and can add tangy flavor to salad dressings and marinades. Although research on the health benefits of ACV after cooking are inconclusive, some people believe it is best to avoid exposing ACV to high temperatures. This process may kill the bacteria in the mother and, especially during a boil, may alter the chemical compound of the acetic acid (an acid that all vinegars are made of). Some cooking is fine—just avoid extreme temperatures to maintain ACV's health benefits. ACV will retain some of its health benefits regardless of whether or not it is heated.

Can ACV be cooked to a certain temperature and retain its health-enhancing enzymes?

Many people drink ACV in hot water with honey or lemon. As long as the water does not reach boiling (212°F) the ACV will maintain its acetic acid. It is unknown what happens to the enzymes, though based on the number of people who drink it this way, warm water does not seem to have a negative impact on the enzymes. To ensure the preservation of the enzymes, drink ACV in room-temperature or lukewarm water. You may also cook with it raw, as in a dressing for a salad.

What health benefits are there to rubbing ACV on your skin?

So far we have been discussing ACV as a drink, but it is also used as a beauty remedy. Diluting the ACV by at least 50 percent is a must, as putting it directly on the skin can be damaging. Once diluted, the ACV and water mixture can be applied with a cotton ball and has a myriad of benefits for skin of all ages. Got acne? No worries. ACV is equipped with antibacterial properties that help treat skin problems and prevent pesky pimples from forming. Got age spots? ACV has alpha hydroxy acids that remove dead skin and reveal the newer, more vibrant layer underneath. Got wrinkles? ACV helps minimize their appearance and keeps skin looking more youthful. Got good skin? Awesome, that's great. ACV can still balance the pH of your skin and keep it glowing.

Is ACV effective for cleaning?

ACV is great for your inner and outer body, and also for the environment. Its antibacterial properties make it a great option for cleaning the kitchen, bathroom, and windows. Diluting ACV with 1 cup of water for every ¼ cup of ACV used will give you an effective cleaning mixture—just put this mix in a spray bottle and get cleaning. You can free up the space under the kitchen sink by replacing other cleaning products with this simple, all-natural, safe, and much cheaper solution. Do not use on stone, however, such as granite countertops, because it may damage the finish.

What essential oils pair well with ACV for health?

Essential oils are a great partner with ACV and offer some great health and beauty benefits. Lavender, peppermint, eucalyptus, rosemary, and lemon essential oils can be mixed with ACV to make deodorants, facial toner, hair rinse, and even bug spray.

How many calories are in 1 teaspoon of ACV?

A great feature of ACV is its low calories. In 1 teaspoon, there is approximately 1 calorie. In 1 tablespoon, there are approximately 3 calories.

What nutrients are in 1 teaspoon of ACV?

One teaspoon of ACV does not contain large quantities of vitamins or minerals. It does have traces of potassium, but it primary benefit is the acetic acid and potentially the proteins and enzymes of the mother. There are traces of iron, sodium, phosphorous, magnesium, manganese, and copper, but their amounts are small. To get the most nutrients out of ACV, use it as a dressing on a nutritious salad.

How much sugar and carbohydrates are in 1 teaspoon of ACV?

There are approximately 0.05 grams of carbohydrates and 0.02 grams of sugar in 1 teaspoon of ACV.

Is there any fat in ACV?

The only fat you will see in ACV is the purported fat-burning properties it has. There is no fat in ACV.

How much potassium and sodium are in 1 teaspoon of ACV? And what health benefits does potassium have?

In 1 teaspoon of ACV, there is almost no sodium and 4 milligrams of potassium. Potassium is one of seven macro minerals that promote healthy body function. It is also an electrolyte that counteracts the sodium in all the salty snacks we consume and maintains healthy blood pressure. Potassium regulates fluid balance and controls the electrical activity of muscles, even the heart. Have you ever been awakened by a painful muscle spasm (sometimes called a charley horse)? This is your body saying, "Hey, give me more potassium." ACV cannot be the sole provider of potassium, but it does contain some to help keep your body functioning properly.

Can ACV be part of an electrolyte recipe?

Move over, energy drinks! ACV is a great ingredient to toss into your homemade electrolyte drink recipe. If you move and sweat, replenishing your electrolytes is a good idea. Electrolytes are substances in our body that help our organs function. Popular ones include sodium and potassium. When we sweat and lose fluid, we also lose electrolytes. The potassium present in ACV makes it a great ingredient for any electrolyte recipe. Adjusting the ingredients for your own personal taste is a must, so do some research and have fun finding the right concoction for you.

What studies have been conducted on the health benefits of ACV?

ACV has a long history of being an effective home remedy for various ailments and supporting overall health. However, the research behind these claims is limited, and more research is needed to scientifically assess the benefits of ACV for our health.

Although more peer-reviewed scientific research studies are needed, some researchers have delved into the murky world of ACV. One study found that ACV may help regulate blood sugar. Men and women with type 2 diabetes drank 2 tablespoons of ACV along with a 1-ounce nibble of cheese before they went to bed. The findings revealed that participants had lower blood sugar levels on the mornings after they ingested the ACV, as compared to eating the same snack without ACV.

Another touted benefit of ACV is its ability to help with weight management. A 2009 study found that when mice were given acetic acid, the primary component of ACV, they developed less body fat than their counterparts who did not consume acetic acid.

Another 2009 study explored the effect of vinegar consumption on body mass index in three separate groups. In the first group, people drank 30 milliliters of vinegar; in the second group, participants consumed 15 milliliters of vinegar; and in the third group, no vinegar was consumed. The results? Both groups that consumed vinegar every day had lower BMIs and weight than those in the group that didn't drink vinegar, suggesting that consuming a small amount of vinegar could lower body weight in people.

So what is the verdict on ACV from a scientific perspective? It's inconclusive—some research provides evidence that ACV is beneficial to health, but not anywhere near the prevalent folk stories told about it. Since there is no way to patent ACV, there is no incentive for corporations to fund the study of it and make money off it. Anyone can produce it and sell it with the appropriate business licenses. This is why natural remedies rarely have a lot of scientific evidence available to support them: because naturally occurring substances cannot be patented. Conversely, when a pharmaceutical formula is invented by a company, it is patented and then studied extensively because of the possibility of making a profit.

Have many times per day is optimal to ingest ACV?

The amount of ACV varies depending on each individual, but generally people take 1 tablespoon diluted in a glass of water 15 minutes before a meal. This means you can take up to 3 tablespoons a day, but only if it feels okay for your body and you have discussed it with your doctor.

How much ACV should you ingest for different ailments?

There is no conclusive evidence on a specific amount being effective for specific issues. As discussed above, ingesting up to 1 tablespoon of ACV diluted in a glass of water three times a day is a range that you can play with and find what works for you. It may take anywhere from 1 to 3 months to notice changes, so patience and monitoring your body and health is key.

What natural sweeteners could you add to ACV beverages to make them taste better?

ACV has a distinct smell and a taste that doesn't fall far from its origin: the apple. Because of these, a bit of sweetener can go a long way. Adding fruit juice can naturally sweeten ACV, or you can opt for maple syrup or, arguably the most popular, honey. Test which hint of sweet tastes the best to you and go with it.

Is it safe to drink ACV straight and undiluted? Why?

It is not safe to drink ACV without diluting it first. A primary ingredient in ACV is acetic acid, which, if ingested regularly without dilution, can be harmful. Although acetic acid is considered weak in comparison to other acids, it can still cause tooth enamel erosion, damage to the esophagus, and even skin burns if not diluted properly. Always err on the side of caution and dilute ACV before consuming it or using it on your skin.

Are apple cider and ACV the same thing?

While both of these great liquids are derived from apples and delicious in their own right, they are very different. Apple cider is made by grinding apples, then straining the pulp produced, and discarding the solids to leave a sweet, satisfying apple drink. ACV goes through a few more processes. The chosen apple pieces are mixed with yeast and fermented, and the bacteria are added to produce the final ACV product.

Are all types of vinegar the same? Do they have the same health benefits?

Not all vinegars are the same. Vinegars are a sour liquid derived from fermenting alcohol and have a pH falling anywhere between 2 and 5. White vinegar is often used in homemade cleaning products and recipes, and balsamic vinegar is commonly used in salad dressings. The British love malt vinegar on their fish and chips, and rice vinegar is found in many Asian recipes. While all vinegars can add great flavor to food, ACV has purported medicinal health benefits that outweigh the others'.

Does ACV have trace amounts of alcohol in it? Can it get you drunk?

The short answer is that any amount of alcohol in ACV is so small that it is negligible. When ACV is being produced, alcohol is fermented into acetic acid, thus changing it from alcohol to acetic acid. Don't worry about getting drunk on ACV—it is not possible.

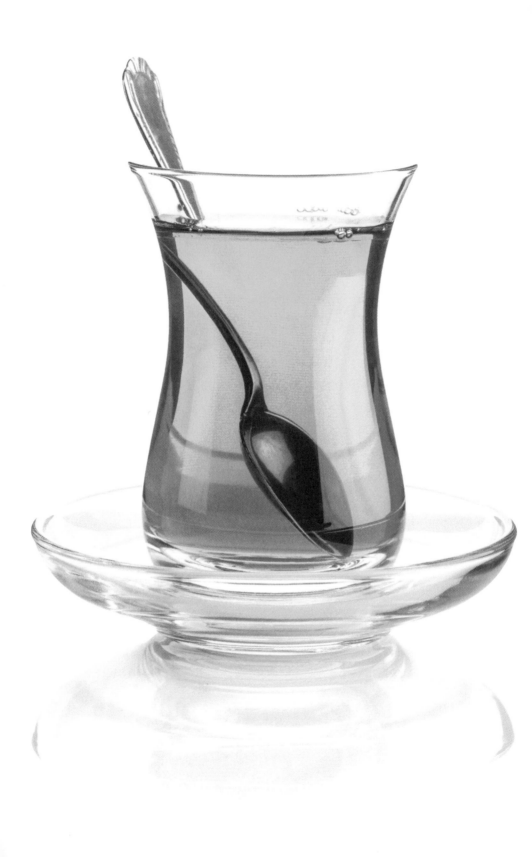

ACKNOWLEDGMENTS

It takes a team of talented professionals to produce a book as beautiful as this. It all started with Lisa Hagan, my incredibly supportive, kind, and savvy literary agent. The team at Sterling is a wonder. Christoper E. Barsanti acquired this book and shepherded it through conception, editing, and eventual release into the world with wise grace and professionalism. Skillful designer Christine Heun created the beautiful visuals you see herein.

As always, I would like to thank my amazing family and friends for all their support and love. I'd also like to thank Karen Nino for making my life easier. Wishing us all radiant health!

GLOSSARY

ACETIC ACID: Vinegar! Its chemical formula is CH_3COOH, and in its pure state it boils at 244.6°F (118.1°C)

ACID: A chemical agent that has a pH lower than 7

ALKALINE: A chemical agent that has a pH higher than 7

ANTIBACTERIAL: Referring to the property of destroying or obstructing the presence of bacteria

ANTIOXIDANT: A substance that hinders the oxidation process

APPLE CIDER VINEGAR: A type of vinegar created from apples and cider

CANDIDA: A type of gut flora that, when overpopulous, can lead to yeast infection and candidiasis

CHLOROGENIC ACID: An acid found in caffeine

CHOLESTEROL: A molecule that is produced by both the human liver and animal-based foods

CONTINUOUS BARREL FERMENTATION METHOD: A process of vinegar making built on the Orleans method, in which a new batch combined new wine with leftover vinegar

DETOXIFY: To remove toxic properties

ENZYME: A biological catalyst that prompts chemical reactions to occur

FERMENTATION: An anaerobic process in which sugar is broken down

GUT MICROBE: A microorganism inhabiting human intestines

INSULIN: A hormone that regulates blood glucose levels

MOTHER OF VINEGAR: A concentration of beneficial bacteria found at the top of ACV

ORLEANS METHOD: A method of crafting vinegar by using oak barrels as fermentation tubs

PATCH TEST: A method of testing a small area of skin with a substance to determine if any irritation occurs

PH: A scale used to measure the acidity or alkalinity of a substance

PHYTOCHEMICAL: Compound found in plants

POSCA: A vinegar tonic consumed by Greeks and Romans

PREBIOTICS: A plant fiber that sustains good bacteria

SWITCHEL: A mixed drink of vinegar, ginger, and water

VINAIGRETTE: A combination of an oil and an acidic substance

VINEGAR: An acidic substance formed by the fermentation of ethanol

PICTURE CREDITS

RESOURCES

BRANDS WE RECOMMEND

Barnes Naturals Organic Apple Cider Vinegar with the Mother

Bragg Organic Apple Cider Vinegar Drink in original, honey, apple-cinnamon, limeade, etc.

Bragg Organic Salad Dressings in original, fat-free, ginger and sesame, pomegranate, etc.

Brandless Organic Raw Apple Cider Vinegar

Dynamic Health Apple Cider Vinegar with Mother

Eden Foods Organic Apple Cider Vinegar

Kevala Organic Raw Apple Cider Vinegar

Spectrum Organic Apple Cider Vinegar with the Mother

Swanson Certified Organic Apple Cider Vinegar with Mother

Vermont Village Organic Apple Cider Vinegar

BOOKS

Patricia Bragg and Paul C. Bragg, *Apple Cider Vinegar: Miracle Health System* (Health Science, 2011).

Sandor Ellix Katz, *The Art of Fermentation: An In-Depth Exploration of Essential Concepts and Processes from Around the World* (Chelsea Green Publishing, 2012).

Paul Pitchford, *Healing with Whole Foods*, 3rd ed. (North Atlantic Books, 2002).

Bettina Malle and Helge Schmickl, *The Artisanal Vinegar Maker's Handbook* (Spikehorn Press, 2015).

Michael Harlan Turkell, *Acid Trip: Travels in the World of Vinegar: With Recipes from Leading Chefs, Insights from Top Producers, and Step-by-Step Instructions on How to Make Your Own* (Abrams, 2017).

WEBSITES

Dr. Axe: www.draxe.com

Bragg: www.bragg.com

The Chopra Center: www.chopra.com

METRIC CONVERSION CHART

US SYSTEM	METRIC SYSTEM
Volume	
1 teaspoon	5 milliliters
1 tablespoon	15 milliliters
¼ cup	60 milliliters
½ cup	120 milliliters
¾ cup	180 milliliters
1 cup	240 milliliters
1 quart	960 milliliters
Weight	
4 ounces	113 grams
8 ounces	227 grams
12 ounces	340 grams
16 ounces	454 grams
Temperature	
300°F	150°C
325°F	160°C
350°F	180°C
375°F	190°C
400°F	200°C
425°F	220°C
450°F	230°C
Baking Pan Size	
8x4x3 inches	20x10x7 centimeters

BIBLIOGRAPHY

"1 Tsp Apple Cider Vinegar." Fat Secret, accessed August 7, 2017. https://www.fatsecret.com/calories-nutrition/usda/vinegar-(cider)?portionid=29657&portionamount=1.000.

"20 Unique Apple Cider Vinegar Uses and Benefits." Dr. Axe, accessed June 29, 2017. https://draxe.com/apple-cider-vinegar-uses.

"3 Major Health Benefits of Apple Cider Vinegar." Primal Source News, accessed October 19, 2017. http://primalsourcenews.com/3-major-health-benefits-of-apple-cider-vinegar.

"3 Reasons Why You Should Use Apple Cider Vinegar for Digestion." CureJoy, accessed October 19, 2017. https://www.curejoy.com/content/apple-cider-vinegar-for-digestion.

"5 Recipes to Get Your Daily Dose of Apple Cider Vinegar." The Healthy Honeys, accessed October 19, 2017. http://thehealthyhoneys.com/5-recipes-drink-apple-cider-vinegar.

"6 Proven Benefits of Apple Cider Vinegar." Authority Nutrition, accessed June 29, 2017. https://authoritynutrition.com/6-proven-health-benefits-of-apple-cider-vinegar.

"6 Proven Benefits of Apple Cider Vinegar." Healthline, accessed October 19, 2017. http://www.healthline.com/nutrition/6-proven-health-benefits-of-apple-cider-vinegar.

"8 Proven Colloidal Silver Benefits, Uses & Side Effects." Dr. Axe, accessed October 19, 2017. https://draxe.com/colloidal-silver-benefits.

"An Apple Cider Vinegar a Day." Good Natural Foods, accessed June 28, 2017. http://www.goodearthnaturlafoods.com.

"Antioxidants, How They Polish Your Life." Health Save Blog, accessed October 19, 2017. https://healthsaveblog.com/antioxidants-how-they-polish-your-life.

"Apple Cider Benefits." Livestrong.com, accessed August 12, 2017. http://www.livestrong.com/article/377670-apple-cider-benefits.

"Apple Cider Health Benefits." Healthy Living Benefits, accessed June 28, 2017. https://www.hlbenefits.com/apple-cider-vinegar-health-benefits.

"Apple Cider Vinegar and Your Health." WebMD, accessed August 7, 2017. http://www.webmd.com/diet/apple-cider-vinegar-and-your-health.

"Apple Cider Vinegar vs. Organic Apple Cider Vinegar." Livestrong.com, accessed August 12, 2017. http://www.livestrong.com/article/107959-apple-cider-vinegar-vs.-organic.

"Can I Clean My House with Apple Cider Vinegar?" SF Gate Home Guides, accessed August 7, 2017. http://homeguides.sfgate.com/can-clean-house-apple-cider-vinegar-104844.html.

"Cancer Statistics." National Institute of Health, accessed July 24, 2017. https://www.cancer.gov/about-cancer/understanding/statistics.

"Cucumber Slaw." All Recipes, accessed October 19, 2017. http://allrecipes.com/video/6536/cucumber-slaw.

"Dandruff." MedBroadcast, accessed October 19, 2017. http://www.medbroadcast.com/condition/getcondition/dandruff.

"Do's and Don'ts of Healing Scar Tissue—Tip #2." Marjorie Brook Seminars, accessed October 19, 2017. http://marjoriebrookseminars.com/tag/treating-open-wounds.

"Does Detoxing Really Help You Lose Weight?" Fit N Fast, accessed July 25, 2017. https://www.fitnfast.com.au/fitness-blog/post/does-detoxing-really-help-you-lose-weight.

"Electrolyte Drinks: Separating the Health from the Hype." A Woman's Health, accessed August 7, 2017. http://awomanshealth.com/electrolyte-drinks-separating-the-health-from-the-hype.

"Essential Oils." Plant Therapy, accessed July 25, 2017. https://www.planttherapy.com.

"Five Home Remedies for Lowering Blood Sugar." Inner Light, accessed June 28, 2017. http://www.inner-light-in.com/2016/04/five-home-remedies-for-lowering-blood-sugar-triglycerides-and-cholesterol.

"Health Benefits of Fermented Foods." Wellness Mama, accessed June 29, 2017. https://wellnessmama.com/2245/fermented-food-benefits.

"Hiatal Hernia." Medicine Net, accessed July 2, 2017. http://www.medicinenet.com/hiatal_hernia_overview/article.htm.

"Home Remedies for Bacterial Vaginosis." Top 10 Home Remedies, accessed August 12, 2017. http://www.top10homeremedies.com/home-remedies/home-remedies-bacterial-vaginosis.html.

"Homemade Organic Raw Apple Cider." Tales of a Kitchen, accessed July 15, 2017. http://talesofakitchen.com/raw/homemade-organic-raw-apple-cider-vinegar.

"How to Make Your Own Kombucha Scoby." The Kitchn, accessed July 13, 2017. http://www.thekitchn.com/how-to-make-your-own-kombucha-scoby-cooking-lessons-from-the-kitchn-202596.

"How to Use APC for Diabetes." Healthy and Natural World, accessed June 28, 2017. http://www.healthyandnaturalworld.com/how-to-use-apple-cider-vinegar-for-diabetes.

"How to Use Apple Cider Vinegar for Vaginal Yeast Infection." Home Remedies, accessed August 12, 2017. http://homeremediesforlife.com/apple-cider-vinegar-for-yeast-infection.

"iHerb Customer Reviews." iHerb, accessed October 19, 2017. https://www.iherb.com/r/Natural-Factors-The-Ultimate-Antioxidant-With-Alpha-Lipoic-Acid-and-Lutein-60-Capsules/2690.

"Is Apple Cider Vinegar a Probiotic?" Livestrong.com, accessed August 12, 2017. http://www.livestrong.com/article/462240-the-benefits-of-apple-cider-vinegar-dosage.

"Mayo Clinic by Mayo Clinic Staff." Mayo Clinic, accessed August 7, 2014. http://www.mayoclinic.org/diseases-conditions/heartburn/basics/definition/con-20019545.

"Medical Definition of PCBs." MedicineNet.com, accessed July 25, 2017. http://www.medicinenet.com/script/main/art.asp?articlekey=19548.

"Migala." Health Magazine, http://www.health.com/health/gallery/0,,20934662,00.html#don-t-give-anything-up-0.

"Mite Infestation Cures." Earth Clinic, accessed October 19, 2017. https://www.earthclinic.com/cures/mite_infestation.html.

"More Info on Detoxification and Cleansing." Organic Nutrition, accessed July 25, 2017. https://www.organicnutrition.co.uk/articles/detoxing-and-cleansing.htm.

"Natural Remedy for Cholesterol." Herbal Daily, accessed June 28, 2017. http://www.herbaldaily.in/natural-remedy-for-cholesterol.html.

"On Regimen in Acute Diseases—The Internet Classics . . .," accessed October 17, 2017. http:/classics.mit.edu/Hippocrates/acutedis.16.16.html.

"On the Articulations." Classics MIT.edu, accessed June 28, 2017. http://classics.mit.edu/Hippocrates/artic.html.

"Organic Food: Sustainable and Healthy Food Production." Eostre Organics, accessed October 6, 2016. http://www.eostreorganics.co.uk/

"Pesticides and Cancer." PubMed.gov, accessed October 10, 2016. https://www.ncbi.nlm.nih.gov/pubmed/9498903

"Probiotics Benefits, Foods and Supplements." Dr. Axe, accessed October 19, 2017. https://draxe.com/probiotics-benefits-foods-supplements.

"Pumpkin Curry Soup." Well Plated, accessed October 19, 2017. www.wellplated.com.

"Research Compares Cost-Effectiveness of Weight-Loss Programs, Drugs." Duke Global Health Institute, accessed July 25, 2017. http://globalhealth. duke.edu/media/news/research-compares-cost-effectiveness-weight-loss-programs-drugs.

"Roman Posca." Romae Vitam, accessed June 28, 2017. http://www.romae-vitam.com/roman-posca.html.

"The Benefits of Apple Cider Vinegar and Dosage." Livestrong.com, accessed August 12, 2017. http://www.livestrong.com/article/462240-the-benefits-of-apple-cider-vinegar-dosage.

"The Internet Classics Archive/On the Articulations by . . .," accessed October 17, 2017. http://classics.mit.edu/Hippocrates/artic.86.86.html.

"The Natural Healing Benefits of Apple Cider Vinegar." Cheyenne Gathering, accessed October 19, 2017. http://cheyennegathering.yuku.com/topic/1017/The-Natural-Healing-Benefits-Of-Apple-Cider-Vinegar.

"The Science of Apple Cider Vinegar." Networx, accessed November 14, 2011. http://www.networx.com/article/the-science-of-vinegar.

"Three Healing Detox Bath Recipes." Wellness Mama, accessed July 25, 2017. https://wellnessmama.com/8331/detox-bath-recipes.

"Use Home Remedies to Quickly and Safely Eliminate Athlete's Foot." Natural News, accessed October 19, 2017. http://www.naturalnews.com/028925_Athletes_foot_home_remedies.html.

"Vaginal pH—Is Your Vagina Acid or Alkaline?" Multi-Gyn, accessed August 12, 2017. https://www.multi-gyn.com/general/vaginal-ph-is-your-vagina-acid-or-alkaline.

"Vinegar Cider, 1-Tsp." Nutritionix, accessed August 7, 2017. https://www.nutritionix.com/i/usda/vinegar-cider-1-tbsp/513fceb375b8dbbc21000286.

"Vinegar History." Enzyme Facts, accessed June 28, 2017. http://www.enzyme-facts.com/vinegar-history.html.

"Vinegar Improves Insulin Sensitivity." American Diabetes Association, accessed June 28, 2017. care.diabetesjournals.org.

"Vinegar: Medicinal Uses and Antiglycemic Effect." NCBI, accessed June 28, 2017. https://www.ncbi.nlm.nih.gov/pmc/articles/PMC1785201.

"What Is Apple Cider Vinegar with the Mother?" Wellness Mama, accessed October 17, 2017. https://wellnessmama.com/121495/apple-cider-vinegar-mother.

"What Visceral Fat Does to the Body." YouTube: The Doctors.

Archer, Jan. "Does Apple Cider Vinegar Lower Blood Pressure?" Livestrong, accessed May 8, 2015. http://www.livestrong.com/article/459624-does-apple-cider-vinegar-lower-blood-pressure.

Axe, Josh. "20 Unique Apple Cider Vinegar Uses and Benefits." Dr. Axe, accessed July 24, 2017. https://draxe.com/apple-cider-vinegar-uses.

Axe, Josh. "Secret Detox Drink Recipe." Dr. Axe, accessed July 25, 2017. https://draxe.com/recipe/secret-detox-drink.

Bauer, Brent A. "What Is BPA, and What Are the Concerns about BPA?" Mayo Clinic, accessed July 25, 2017. http://www.mayoclinic.org/healthy-lifestyle/nutrition-and-healthy-eating/expert-answers/bpa/faq-20058331.

Bright, Sierra. "5 Reasons to Wash Your Face and Skin with Apple Cider Vinegar." Natural Living Ideas, accessed December 14, 2015. http://www.naturallivingideas.com/5-reasons-to-wash-your-face-with-apple-cider-vinegar.

Brusco, Jessica. "Recommended Amount of Apple Cider Vinegar Per Day." Livestrong, accessed April 22, 2015. http://www.livestrong.com/article/494866-recommended-amount-of-apple-cider-vinegar-per-day.

Bruso, Jessica. "Does Drinking Apple Cider Vinegar Affect Your Body's pH?" Livestrong, accessed October 19, 2017. http://www.livestrong.com/article/531375-does-drinking-apple-cider-vinegar-affect-your-bodys-ph.

Campbell, Susan. "The Most Delicious Electrolyte Drink." Chef Teton Essential Cuisine, accessed August 25, 2015. http://susanteton.com/blog/the-most-delicious-electrolyte-drink.

Collins, Sonya. "Alkaline Diets," WebMD, accessed October 19, 2017. http://www.webmd.com/diet/a-z/alkaline-diets.

Gorsky, Faith. "Healthy Peanut Butter, Banana, and Honey Milkshake." An Edible Mosaic, accessed July 25, 2017. http://www.anediblemosaic.com/healthy-peanut-butter-banana-honey-milkshake.

Han, Emily. "Recipe: Quinoa and Black Bean Salad with Orange-Coriander Dressing." The Kitchn, accessed July 25, 2017. http://www.thekitchn.com/recipe-quinoa-and-black-bean-salad-with-orange-coriander-dressing-recipes-from-the-kitchn-182318.

Hills, Jenny. "How to Use Apple Cider Vinegar for Weight Loss." Healthy and Natural World, accessed July 25, 2017. http://www.healthyandnaturalworld.com/how-to-use-apple-cider-vinegar-for-weight-loss.

Johns, Audrey. "Strawberry Blueberry ACV Detox Smoothie." Lose Weight by Eating, accessed July 25, 2017. https://www.loseweightbyeating.com/apple-cider-vinegar-detox-drink-recipes.

Johnston, C. S., and A. J. Buller. "Vinegar and Peanut Products as Complementary Foods to Reduce Postprandial Glycemia." *Journal of the American Dietetic Association* 105, no. 12 (2005): 1939–1942, accessed October 19, 2017. https://www.ncbi.nlm.nih.gov/pubmed/16321601.

Johnston, C. S., and C. A. Gaas. "Vinegar: Medicinal Uses and Antiglycemic Effect." *Medscape General Medicine* 8, no. 2 (2006): 61.

Johnston, Carol S., Cindy M. Kim, and Amanda J. Buller. "Vinegar Improves Insulin Sensitivity to a High-Carbohydrate Meal in Subjects with Insulin Resistance or Type 2 Diabetes." *Diabetes Care* 27, no. 1 (2004): 281–282, accessed October 19, 2017. http://care.diabetesjournals.org/content/27/1/281.long.

Kimball, Molly. "Apple Cider Vinegar: Sorting through Fact and Fiction." NOLA, accessed September 29, 2014. http://www.nola.com/healthy-eating/2014/09/apple_cider_vinegar_fact_and_f.html.

Kondo, Tomoo, et al. "Acetic Acid Upregulates the Expression of Genes for Fatty Acid Oxidation Enzymes in Liver to Suppress Body Fat Accumulation." *Journal of Agricultural and Food Chemistry* 57, no. 13 (2009): 5982–5986.

Kondo, Tomoo, et al. "Vinegar Intake Reduces Body Weight, Body Fat Mass, and Serum Triglyceride Levels in Obese Japanese Subjects." *Bioscience, Biotechnology, and Biochemistry* 73, no. 8 (2009): 1837–1843.

Leech, Joe. "The Alkaline Diet: An Evidence-Based Review." Healthline, accessed October 19, 2017. https://www.healthline.com/nutrition/the-alkaline-diet-myth.

Loux, Renee. "9 Ways to Use Vinegar for More Beautiful Skin and Hair." Women's Health, accessed October 19, 2017. http://www.womenshealthmag.com/beauty/beauty-uses-for-vinegar.

Marshal, Paul. "Vinegar and Calcium Absorption." Livestrong, accessed October 19, 2017. http://www.livestrong.com/article/286934-vinegar-calcium-absorption.

Mercola, Joseph. "What the Research Really Says about Apple Cider Vinegar." Mercola, accessed October 19, 2017. http://articles.mercola.com/sites/articles/archive/2009/06/02/apple-cider-vinegar-hype.aspx.

Mitrou, Panayota, et al. "Vinegar Consumption Increases Insulin-Stimulated Glucose Uptake by the Forearm Muscle in Humans with Type 2 Diabetes." *Journal of Diabetes Research* (2015), accessed June 28, 2017. https://www.ncbi.nlm.nih.gov/pmc/articles/PMC4438142.

Niall, Alana. "Apple Cider Vinegar Salad." HubPages, accessed July 25, 2017. https://hubpages.com/food/Apple-Cider-Vinegar-Recipes.

Ostman, E., et. al. "Vinegar Supplementation Lowers Glucose and Insulin Responses and Increases Satiety after a Bread Meal in Healthy Subjects." *European Journal of Clinical Nutrition* 59, no. 9 (2005): 983–988, accessed October 19, 2017. https://www.ncbi.nlm.nih.gov/pubmed/16015276.

Perkins, Sabrina. "5 Natural Ways to Get Rid of Dandruff." Naturally Curly, accessed October 19, 2017. https://www.naturallycurly.com/curlreading/ingredients/5-natural-ways-to-get-rid-of-dandruff-si.

Rettner, Rachael. "Some Weight Loss Supplements Contain Amphetamine-Like Compound." Live Science, accessed July 25, 2017. https://www.livescience.com/41336-weight-loss-supplements-acacia-rigidula.html.

Ryan, Charlene. "pH Acidity/Alkaline Balance Foods." Livestrong, accessed October 19, 2017. http://www.livestrong.com/article/433498-ph-acidity-alkaline-balance-foods.

Schwalfenberg, Gerry K. "The Alkaline Diet: Is There Evidence That an Alkaline pH Diet Benefits Health?" *Journal of Environmental and Public Health* 2012 (2012), accessed October 19, 2017. https://www.hindawi.com/journals/jeph/2012/727630.

Shirazi, Sylvie. "Shaved Golden Beet, Carrot and Radish Salad with Coriander Mustard Vinaigrette." Gormande in the Kitchen, accessed July 25, 2017. http://gourmandeinthekitchen.com/shaved-beet-carrot-radish-salad-recipe.

Solieri, Laura, and Paolo Guidici, eds. *Vinegars of the World*: Springer, 2009.

Spiegel, Allison. "A Guide to Where Your Vinegar Comes From and How to Use It." Huffington Post, accessed March 27, 2012. http://www.huffingtonpost.com/2014/11/24/vinegar-guide_n_1380713.htm.

Spritzler, Franziska. "7 Side Effects of Too Much Apple Cider Vinegar." Health Line, accessed August 10, 2016. http://www.healthline.com/nutrition/apple-cider-vinegar-side-effects#section3.

Stöppler, Melissa Conrad. "Yeast Infection (in Women and Men)." MedicineNet.com, accessed August 12, 2017. http://www.medicinenet.com/yeast_infection_in_women_and_men/article.htm.

Thompson, Jennifer. "Benefits of Raw Apple Cider Vinegar." Healthy Bliss, accessed October 19, 2017. http://healthybliss.net/benefits-of-raw-apple-cider-vinegar.

Vaughn, Karen. "What's the Story about Vinegar and Probiotics?". Acupuncture Brooklyn, accessed July 26, 2012. http://www.acupuncturebrooklyn.com/alternative-health/whats-the-story-about-vinegar-and-probiotics.

Ware, Megan. "Potassium: Health Benefits, Recommended Intake." Medical News Today, accessed December 16, 2016. http://www.medicalnewstoday.com/articles/287212.php.

Way, Jason, ND. "How and Where Your Body Stores Toxins." Curebiome Naturopathic, accessed July 25, 2017. http://www.curebiome.com/how-and-where-your-body-stores-toxins.

White, Andrea M., and C. S. Johnston. "Vinegar Ingestion at Bedtime Moderates Waking Glucose Concentrations in Adults with Well-Controlled Type 2 Diabetes." *Diabetes Care* 30, no. 11 (2007): 2814–2815.

Wilcox, Julie. "7 Benefits of Quinoa: The Supergrain of the Future." *Forbes*, accessed October 19, 2017. https://www.forbes.com/sites/juliewilcox/2012/06/26/7-benefits-of-quinoa-the-supergrain-of-the-future.

Wolf, Naomi. *The Beauty Myth* (New York: HarperPerennial, 2002).

INDEX

Note: Page numbers in *italics* indicate recipes.

ABOUT THE AUTHOR

Amy Leigh Mercree's motto is "Live joy. Be kind. Love unconditionally." She counsels women and men in the underrated art of self-love to create happier lives. Amy is a best-selling author, media personality, and medical intuitive. Mercree speaks internationally, focusing on compassion, joy, and wellness.

Mercree is the best-selling author of eight books, including *The Spiritual Girl's Guide to Dating: Your Enlightened Path to Love, Sex, and Soul Mates*; *A Little Bit of Chakras: An Introduction to Energy Healing*; *Joyful Living: 101 Ways to Transform Your Spirit and Revitalize Your Life*; *The Chakras and Crystals Cookbook: Juices, Sorbets, Smoothies, Salads, and Crystal Infusions to Empower Your Energy Centers*; *The Compassion Revolution: 30 Days of Living from the Heart*; *A Little Bit of Meditation*; and *The Holistic Guide to Essential Oils*.

Mercree has been featured in *Glamour, Women's Health, Inc., Shape, The Huffington Post, Your Tango, Soul and Spirit Magazine*, and MindBodyGreen, and on NBC, CBS, and many more media outlets.

Check out AmyLeighMercree.com for articles, picture quotes, and quizzes. Mercree is fast becoming one of the most quoted women on the web. See what all the buzz is about.

@AmyLeighMercree on Twitter, Snapchat, and Instagram.

＊

To download your free apple cider vinegar and essential oils tool kit and power up your health and vitality right now, go to www.amyleighmercree.com/oilandvinegartoolkit and use password OILandVINEGAR.